Country Folk Medicine

COUNTRY FOLK MEDICINE

Tales of Skunk Oil, Sassafras Tea, and Other Old-Time Remedies

gathered by
Elisabeth Janos

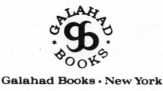

Galahad Books · New York

First Galahad Books edition published in 1995.

Galahad Books
A division of Budget Book Service, Inc.
386 Park Avenue South
New York, NY 10016

Galahad Books is a registered trademark of Budget Book Service, Inc.

Published by arrangement with The Globe Pequot Press.

Library of Congress Catalog Card Number: 90-42571

ISBN: 0-88365-903-4

Printed in the United States of America.

For Mother, Heather Lyn Janos, and Bonnie Rae

Contents

Introduction

Curious about old-time medicinal self-treatment in rural and semirural New England and New York State, I decided in the winter of 1983 to go straight to the horse's mouth. My plan was to keep interviewing senior citizens until I had a well-rounded picture of this aspect of the past. I had no idea how enormous the task would be.

Experience soon taught me that the most expedient way to gather material was to drop into senior centers two or three hours before the lunch program began. Sometimes I got to the centers before the people I wanted to interview.

I was never refused entry to any center, and the people were always gracious and often eager to talk with me. In fact, the topic often got the conversation rolling, and sometimes as I moved on to another person or group of people, I could still hear tales about old-time medicine being discussed by the people I had just interviewed.

In the afternoons, I visited nursing homes. Some barred my entry due to rights-of-privacy laws. Nonetheless when granted entry, I encountered the same enthusiasm and good will.

I asked people what they had used to treat themselves, as well as what their parents had used on them. There were folks who had always relied on doctors and had no remedies to give me. Some claimed to have been healthy all their lives; others couldn't remember that far back. Some of those who did remember turned up a wealth of information. A general picture began to emerge.

For four and a half years, I traveled at every opportunity. Eventually, I spoke to more than 3,000 people; about 1,400 of them were able to provide me with remedies they had used—more than 7,000 recipes, procedures, and recommendations. Finally, I realized that even if the research continued for the rest of my life, I would still have more to learn. At the same time, I felt I had become thoroughly familiar with the most widely credited treatments.

The scope of this project has been limited to natural substances. Often, they were general household staples. For isolated people, it was especially important to use healing substances that were within arm's reach. Some products were purchased from the general store or pharmacy, but I have included only those that were bought in pure form; this project does not cover patent medicine. The reader will find much cross-referencing of material: Often, the same basic products were used for many different conditions.

There were no hard-and-fast rules as to quantities of medicinal substances used, as measuring was not as fashionable as it is today; "a pinch," "a dab," or "a small handful" might be part of the formula. When discussing quantities, I have cited the general consensus.

The book opens with a chapter titled "Some Unusual Healing Substances." This chapter addresses products that were an integral part of Yankee folk medicine that may appear both bizarre and unwholesome today. I hope this overview will give the reader a better understanding of the more peculiar materials used.

In the rest of the book, the remedies are grouped in chapters according to physical problems; included are the most popular remedies for each condition. At the end of each section, other approaches are listed: these were remedies that were employed with some frequency, yet were not standard. Also included are remedies that I felt were particularly significant or interesting.

There will be different reactions from different readers: Some will find a great deal of humor in the following pages, while others will be appalled and even disgusted. Surely there will be some who give our grandparents a great share of credit for many of the commonsense remedies that were used at the turn of the century and well into the 1900s. Indeed, several of the treatments persist to this day.

WHEN DOCTORS WERE SCARCE

At the turn of the century, few medical schools existed, so there was a shortage of licensed physicians. When World War I broke out, many of the existing medical personnel rallied to the cause and joined the service, leaving their patients to fend for themselves.

Many of the doctors that were available were of the "down-home" variety, and they often practiced a mixture of allopathic and folk medicine. Women might be told to wait for the full moon to wean a baby; a salt pork poultice might be prescribed for an infection; or a mustard plaster might be applied to relieve congestion.

The following story was told to me by a 103-year-old lady from Greenfield, Massachusetts.

Everybody went to school in the same school. The teacher let my brother out about half an hour before the rest of us because it was his first year. He took our dinner pail, put it on the stone wall under the trees, and took out a sandwich. He forgot to put the pail cover on.

I was the oldest, so when I went out, I divided our lunches, and we ate our sandwiches. And there was a piece of apple pie for each of us. I bit into my piece and there was a hornet in it that stung my lip. I was allergic to them, and my face began to swell. And the teacher couldn't stop it; so she took my aunt, five years older than me, who was in the same room, and had her take me home. She made me run part of the way. By the time I got home, my face was swollen sore, and I could hardly see out of my eye.

So they rushed me to the doctor and he said there wasn't anything he could do. He said to take a plantain leaf from the yard, roll it, and put it on my face. That took it down by the time I went to bed. That was havin' to doctor-by-guess.

There were other ways as well in which the medical profession was vastly different than it is today. As one of my informants related,

The doctor came to your house in those days, in the middle of the night or anytime. A home visit was a dollar. For that money, the doctor would check out anyone in the family that was sick. When it got to be two dollars, Mother thought that was outrageous.

People spoke of being extremely poor in their early years. In rural areas there was little industry; consequently, making a living was often difficult. As an added complication, families tended to be quite large; it could be a challenge to keep everyone fed and clothed. In 1929, the Depression struck with a vengeance; for many, it added to an already severe burden. Frequently, a doctor was not called in unless illness threatened life. The indigent sometimes bartered for medical treatment, usually with whatever they could spare.

When it came to sickness, with twelve kids, my mother had to know the answer. When we had to have the doctor, he got paid whatever we had—potatoes, pork, ham—we smoked our own ham and bacon in a little house out back. In the root cellar we had turnips, carrots, and beets. Sometimes she dressed chickens to give to the doctor for trade.

Services were also traded for medical attention:

Dad got hurt and couldn't work for a year. They were clearing rocks off a field and were putting them in a wagon. On the rig there was a staff that went through the middle between two horses, and Papa was on the stick fixing the horses' collar.

The first automobile in town came by, and the man honked his horn. The horses reared and galloped away. Papa fell between the two horses and got run over by them. One stepped on his knee; he had a broken leg. Mother did housework for the doctor in exchange for his services.

Not only were doctors different in our grandparents' time, but being sick was vastly different from the way it is today. If there was a dwelling with a dangerous, contagious disease within, extreme measures were taken—a large red quarantine sign was posted on the front door, and no one was allowed to enter or leave. One woman described this practice.

> *The quarantine sign was put up by the doctor, the Board of Health,*
> *or the Overseer of the Poor (they were in charge of poor people, charity).*
> *If you wanted food, it would be delivered outside your house. It made you*
> *feel like you had leprosy or something.*

In some homes, the quarantine was carried a step further; sick people were sent to their rooms for the duration of the illness and not allowed to mingle with family members. One woman recalled the time her mother had the flu; they would open the door a crack and push food into her room. Another told about the time her sister had chicken pox: "I wasn't supposed to go in her room, but I did. Then I had to stay in there with her. I caught them and was in her room for three weeks."

A woman from Gloucester, Massachusetts, told how schools and hospitals were also strict about quarantine.

> *I was in the hospital in Lynn when I had scarlet fever. In school, they*
> *burned my books and everything in my desk, and sprayed my desk. I was*
> *in the hospital on the second floor, and my father took a ladder and climbed*
> *up and showed me the doll he was going to give me when I got out. I'd*
> *never had a doll before in my life.*

Country folk did not yield to illness without putting up a fight. Sometimes, even the threat of illness was enough to elicit action.

> *My sister was awful sick with smallpox and Aunt Mary was afraid*
> *I'd get it too. She took a piece of broken glass, sterilized it with a match,*
> *and cut my arm. She took a scab from my sister and pressed it into the*
> *cut. I didn't get smallpox, so maybe the vaccination "took."*

At other times, people were helpless in the face of disease; folk medicine gave little or no relief. Such was the case in 1918, when a new strain of flu seemed to come out of nowhere. In its wake, it left an estimated 20,000,000 people dead throughout the world. Everyone was panicky and people kept their distance from others. The family unit was often dramatically changed overnight.

One woman told how she used to stand and look out the window and see the horse-drawn hearses bringing bodies to the cemetery all day long. Another said, "It was the real flu, it wasn't the imitation you have today. You didn't feel good one day, the next day you were in bed, and the third day you were dead." A soldier who had returned from Brest related that people there died so fast that they couldn't do anything but stack them up.

A man from a small New Hampshire town remembered an incident from that infamous year.

> I'll never forget when we stopped in at one house on the way to school. We were coming down the old road. Mr. Powers was driving the sleigh, and he said we'd better stop in and see why the fire wasn't going. There were five people in the house and they were all dead. Three of them were kids. We had to go to Bangor to get the coffins, because the undertaker couldn't keep up. Pregnant women got hit real hard.

DID FOLK MEDICINE WORK?

When we look at old-time remedies, it's hard in some cases to draw a line between medicine and magic. Did a piece of red cloth tied around the neck really prevent nosebleeds? Did a dishrag rubbed on a wart and then buried in the ground really cure that common skin affliction? In other instances, folk wisdom has been proved valid. For example, cod-liver oil was taken by many in the cold-weather months to prevent infections. In the past few years, research on fish oil has flourished, and it is now known that certain fish oils boost the immune system in a number of ways due to their high concentration of vitamin A.

Many other of the home remedies our grandparents relied on are still in use in some form or another. Wintergreen oil, which was applied externally to give temporary relief from rheumatic complaints, contains an aspirinlike compound called methyl salicylate. This substance is still a popular ingredient in many over-the-counter preparations for aches and pains. Similarly, cloves and clove oil, which were used to numb the pain of a toothache, contain a substance called eugenol, a product that dentists have been using for years as a local anesthetic.

Many of the elders I spoke with described taking a sulfur-and-molasses tonic in spring. The use of sulfur in medicine goes back to the ancient Chinese and Egyptians. Today's sulfa drugs were developed based on sulfur research. With the advent of sulfa drugs, allopathic medicine—traditional medicine as we know it—became firmly established, then later bloomed when penicillin became widely used.

Certain animal oils were very popular, used both internally and externally. I heard many stories of bringing children out of life-threatening respiratory conditions with such substances. For instance, chicken fat was used to treat croup, colds, and pneumonia. Chicken soup has been shown to be a mild expectorant, although the active ingredient has not been identified. Perhaps the chicken fat itself is responsible. In any case, certain oils appear to regulate moisture at the cellular level, as well as providing concentrated fuel for metabolic processes. Today, doctors warn us that it is dangerous to put infants and toddlers on a low-fat diet, for many types of infections can result.

Our elders used manure and urine to treat a host of complaints. While we shake our heads in horror at the use of "sewage pharmacology," in fact it is still in use today. Many women are familiar with a hormone prescription called premarin: its manufacture calls for pregnant mares' urine. *E. coli*, a bacterium normally found in feces, comes in handy in labs where insulin, interferon, or interleukin is genetically engineered.

We cannot say why the use of mud neutralized insect stings, but antibiotics such as Aureomycin, streptomycin, Terramycin, cyclosporine, and nystatin come from microbes in the soil.

Some Yankee folk remedies share a venerable history. *The Papyrus Ebers,* thought to be the oldest surviving book in the world,[1] is filled with medical remedies reminiscent of those our grandparents relied on.

Examples include flax, sulfur, castor oil, olive oil, goose fat, aloe, fennel, garlic, peppermint, salt, milk, alum, onions, turpentine, wormwood, and urine and excrement. An Egyptian recipe for pain in the abdomen includes peppermint in its formula; one for earache calls for olive oil; a remedy for constipation includes castor beans. Similar remedies can be found in this book.

Readers should draw their own conclusions as to why some of these remedies have survived for more than 3,000 years.

---

[1] Cyril P. Bryan, *The Papyrus Ebers* (London: Garden City Press, 1930).

- 1 -

Some Unusual Healing Substances

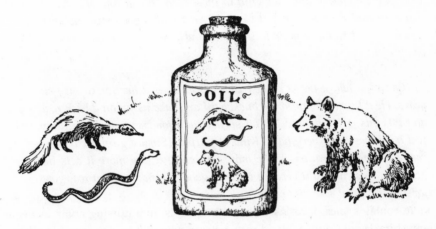

RESINS AND TURPENTINE

Perhaps as far back as the stone age, our ancestors observed that, when certain types of trees are injured, they produce a sticky substance that forms a seal over the wound. The first medicinal applications of resins were probably on injuries similar to those incurred by trees—cuts and wounds.

In ancient Egypt, numerous medicinal formulas included the gum-resin myrrh, a product that exudes from abrasions in the bark of small trees of the genus *Commiphora*. The use of resins has persisted throughout recorded history: In modern times, physicians still take advantage of their curative properties.

Senior citizens sometimes spoke of chewing the resin "spruce gum"; this was the precursor of our modern chewing gum. After it is chewed for a while, it is remarkably similar to store-bought gum—except for the strong pine flavor and firmer texture. A few cited medicinal reasons for its use, but usually they chewed it just for the pleasure of it.

I've chewed spruce gum countless times. This was found only on our native spruce, which I believe is the white spruce. When the bark on the spruce tree is badly bruised, the pitch runs out and, after quite a length of time, hardens and cures into a hard resin. We would take a jackknife and pry it off the tree.

———

Take a large lump of spruce gum and chew it—just tastes good. That's all we had; didn't have gum in those days. It's yellow. It's the sap that runs and hardens; when it bleeds, it comes up a good-size bubble. It was supposed to make your teeth white and clean, and it was good for bad breath.

———

Grandpa had a horse named Black Beauty, had her for twenty-six years. He'd hitch her up to the buckboard and take us up on a back road and take his jackknife and cut off spruce gum for chewing. It's a lump, real hard, has to be very hard. Kind of purple. [Spruce gum occurs in a range of light colorations.] The more you chew it, the more it acts like gum. Us kids chewed it because it tastes good; Grandpa said it was good for digestion and sour stomach.

Folklore contains tales of resins curing tuberculosis. In a nursing home in Keene, New Hampshire, I spoke with a retired navy veteran who told me she "was in for life."

When I was fifteen, I had galloping consumption [tuberculosis]; I was weak all the time and couldn't get enough air. The doctors weren't able to help me, so I was sent to Grandpa's farm to recover. He would take a pint of gin and add spruce gum and shake the hell out of it until it emulsified. When you shake it well, it gets like Scott's Emulsion. It would make a sticky liquid, kind of like a white paste. He faithfully gave me a tablespoon of it every four hours; and in several months I was cured.

In the section on piles, I've discussed resinous substances that were used to treat this irksome condition. Piles and stomach ulcers sometimes occur simultaneously; resins were also sometimes used to treat ulcers. A retired druggist told me that an old friend of his used to swallow pitch by the spoonful for a stomach ulcer. I was given the following remedy, which also contains resin:

For bleeding ulcers: In the spring, break off branches from the tama-rack tree and peel off the bark. Cut up the bark and simmer it. Place it in a jar and put it in the refrigerator. Take one tablespoon before each meal.

The semiprecious gem amber is a fossil resin found in alluvial soil; three people recalled its use for a thyroid problem. I received the following account from a lady in Worcester, New York:

My mother-in-law had swollen glands, bulging eyes; she'd get out of breath: a thyroid problem. She suffered from age thirty to fifty-eight or sixty, about thirty years. She bought real amber beads, wore them like a choker, close to the neck. In a while, her symptoms went away. She had such a belief in that, she wore it day and night for the rest of her life. Never took it off except when she had a bath. Never complained anymore after that.

Very few seniors were familiar with balm of Gilead, which was made from the resin of balsam poplar buds. However, the people who had used it spoke highly of it. It was used as a liniment for sprains, bruises, sores, rheumatism, and aches and pains.

I spoke with a very short little man who had curly snow-white hair and thick glasses.

Every spring I would go with Grandmother and pick Gilead buds off a tree. Grandfather would go to the bar and get a pint of alcohol. We'd put a bunch of the buds in a jar and pour alcohol over them. In a day or two we'd strain the buds out. It was an all-around liniment.

A chipper lady who writes children's stories told me that I could find a "Gilead tree" on her old homestead, a place called Tiny Farm. When I left her apartment, I headed into the country, and a winding road brought me to the location. I knocked on her grandson's door and was given permission to pick some of the buds: it was April and they were just starting to open.

The first thing I noticed was that the buds exude a peculiar odor. To me, they smelled like sweet medicine; a few people commented that they smelled like turpentine. When I started to pick the buds, a sticky resin rubbed off on my hands. When I got home, I put the buds in a jar of rubbing alcohol. A few minutes later I noticed that the solution had turned brown—much of the resin had been drawn out that rapidly.

The medical profession also used resinous substances on a myriad of complaints. Old volumes of *materia medica* and old pharmacopoeias abound with such items: balsam of Canada (from the balsam fir); burgundy pitch (from spruce fir); hemlock pitch (from the hemlock spruce); Venice turpentine (a resin from the larch tree); Peruvian balsam (from a tropical American tree); and balsam of tolu (from a South American tree).

• • •

When pitch is vaporized and condensed through distillation, it becomes the common turpentine with which we are all familiar. In many cases, turpentine was used externally, either straight or in combination with one or more other substances, to keep it from burning the skin.

When I was beginning this project, I was shocked to learn that a few drops of turpentine had sometimes been placed on a teaspoon of sugar and ingested for medicinal reasons, such as for worms, a sore throat, or a cold. The sugar on which the turpentine was dropped was an effective vehicle, for it served as a buffer and also guaranteed rapid absorption into the bloodstream.

In my research, I have noticed that a few modern authors have stated incorrectly that common turpentine was never taken internally. This is an easy mistake to make because old writers labeled *sap* from certain trees as turpentine. Adding to the confusion, we find several different labels on common turpentine. In a contemporary work on toxicology, we learn, "Turpentine, gum turpentine, oil of turpentine, and spirits of turpentine are essentially synonymous names."[1]

Several years ago I was surprised to find one bottle of gum spirits of turpentine in our local drugstore. The label warned, "For external use only."

In a book called *The Medical Repository*, published in 1821, I found a lengthy article by a Dr. Samuel Osborn. The chapter is devoted solely to the internal and external use of spirits of turpentine; its effectiveness is cited for use in over a dozen maladies, some of which were life-threatening. Among Osborn's remarks: spirit of turpentine "was an article of the *materia medica*, and in great repute, more than two centuries ago. . . . It is not to be expected that any medicine will operate more powerfully than this does. . . . For my own part, I have never obtained the knowledge of a single fact from books, or conversation, or my own observations that any serious inconvenience, or any permanent injury, ever resulted from the discreet use of this valuable remedy. What may be justly said of this can hardly be said with truth of any other very powerful medicine."[2]

Doctors continued to administer turpentine well into the present century; however, they became increasingly aware of side effects. *The Modern Home Physician*, published in 1939, states, "Turpentine is sometimes used in half-ounce doses, with an equal quantity of castor oil, as a means of killing and dislodging tapeworms, but there is a risk of giving turpentine inwardly as it may cause severe inflammation of the kidneys with the appearance of large quantities of albumin and blood in the urine."[3]

Another source states the symptoms of an overdose: "There is a strong odor of turpentine in the breath, and any urine that is passed may smell of violets. . . . Breathing is embarrassed and noisy. There may be collapse and convulsions. In some cases great pain is experienced."[4]

A modern book on toxicology gives a general indication of fatal dosage. "As little as 15 ml. (one-half ounce) has proved fatal to a child . . . but a few children have survived 2 and even 3 oz. . . . The mean lethal dose in adults probably lies between 4 and 6 oz."[5]

[1] Robert E. Gosselin, M.D., Ph.D., and Harold C. Hodge, Ph.D., D.Sc., et al. *Clinical Toxicology of Commercial Products.* (Baltimore: Williams and Wilkins, 1977), p. 315.

[2] Samuel L. Mitchill, M.D.; James R. Manley, M.D.; Felix Pascalis, M.D.; Charles Drake, M.D. *The Medical Repository on Original Essays and Intelligence,* vol. 6. (New York: William A. Mercein, 1821), p. 394–98.

[3] Victor Robinson, Ph.C., M.D., ed., *The Modern Home Physician* (New York: William H. Wise and Co., 1939), pp. 734–35.

[4] J. L. Corish, M.D., ed. *Health Knowledge,* vol. 2 (New York: Domestic Health Society, 1924), p. 1102.

[5] Gosselin et. al., op.cit., p. 315.

The following story demonstrates that turpentine fumes pose a threat to infants. It was told by a lady in a nursing home in Newport, Vermont, whose skin was dappled with brown age spots. She was born in 1892, but her mind was evidently clear as crystal.

I lost my three-month-old daughter in May when they were painting the house. It was a warm day and I had all the windows open for air. The night before, she was perfectly all right; when I checked her about 3:00 A.M., she was fine. When I got up at 5:00 o'clock she was breathing funny; it was almost like she wasn't breathing at all. I called the neighbor and the neighbor called the doctor; by the time he got there, she had passed away.

After she expired, she purged three times from the mouth and nose; the vomit was a greenish color and it smelled like turpentine. Paint used to come with turpentine in it, and the doctor thought that's what killed her.

Turpentine was used in the past to induce abortions, and my research leads me to conclude that pregnant women should stay clear of even the fumes of this substance. One source told me, "A lot of women got ruined from taking it. They would keep on taking it until they would abort and burn their insides out."

KEROSENE

Kerosene is distilled from petroleum, which is a naturally occurring oil that comes from under the ground. Yankees learned to use petroleum from the Indians: certain tribes procured the substance in western New York State and western Pennsylvania.

In the 1700s a missionary "classed `Fossil oil' as one of the favorite medicines of the Indians. Besides its use in external complaints of all sorts, he reported that it would burn in a lamp and that the Indians sold it to white people at four guineas a quart."[6]

When kerosene was first refined in the 1850s, it began to supplant the heavier oil. Kerosene, which was also called coal oil, was used in the same manner as turpentine: A few drops were placed on a teaspoon of sugar and ingested. Occasionally it was taken in much larger dosage; some people took as much as a full ounce, but this was not common. Kerosene was ingested more often than turpentine; but, unlike turpentine, it was not often used externally except for head lice.

Before the days of electric lights, kerosene lamps were widely used, and kerosene had to be refined well to cut down on the smoke produced by lamps. Many seniors told

---

[6] Virgil J. Vogel, *American Indian Medicine* (Norman: University of Oklahoma Press, 1970), p. 403. In the 1800s, another missionary extolled its external virtues and added, "Some also take it internally and it appears to have hurt no one in this way."[7]

[7] Ibid., p. 402.

me they would not take the kerosene that is on the market today because it is not refined well. Said one:

Today's kerosene is poison, it's like the type C bunker oil we used to get. I wouldn't dare take it now. It used to be clear kerosene then; it was pure.

Although kerosene was most commonly used for sore throats, colds, and croup, it was believed to be effective for a variety of ailments.

Old Doctor Thomas gave the Pratt boy up for dead because he had pneumonia so bad. His father and mother were up all night giving him a few drops of kerosene on sugar every so often. In the morning his lungs were clear.

—

My son slept in a rickety bed. When I would hear the bed shaking, I'd know right away what was wrong: he'd be having convulsions. I would give him kerosene on a teaspoon of sugar and it would stop the convulsions.

—

Kerosene cured our family of black diphtheria. The mouth and throat filled with a white foamy material. Dump some kerosene out of a lamp and swab the throat with it. It would cut it and clean it out.

—

When my ears got frostbitten, I rubbed kerosene on them. When I got to the doctor, he told me it was the best thing I could have done.

—

Johnny Bell used to deliver oil in a horse and buggy. He'd take a little sip of kerosene every so often as a tonic; he lived to be almost a hundred years old.

A lady in a nursing home in Freeport, Maine, gave me some veterinary pointers concerning kerosene. As she spoke, she sat erect on the side of the bed, and rocked thoughtfully back and forth.

Kerosene is a sure cure for fowl. Years ago, we had an infection in one of our five henhouses. You put on different rubbers each time you go into another henhouse, so the contamination doesn't spread.

Take an empty tin can, something you can dispose of afterwards. Put kerosene in it. Pull out a small feather of the chicken—you have to be careful though, because it hurts them. Grab a chicken by the leg, stretch the neck, and open the mouth. Dip the tip of the feather in regular fuel kerosene; take the feather and put a few drops down the chicken's throat.

The chickens would be fine the next day. They never died.

For humans, the greatest danger of taking a small dose of kerosene, such as a few drops on a teaspoon of sugar, was that the substance would accidentally be breathed into the lungs, where it could cause serious damage or even death.

SKUNK OIL

Skunk oil, rendered from skunk fat, was one of the more popular healing substances used by our grandparents in the Northeast, reportedly because it had better "penetrating powers" and "staying properties" than most of the other oils that were used. A few people claimed that when you rubbed skunk oil on your hand, you could feel it go through to the other side.

Did skunk oil smell? I got mixed answers on this one. Many said it had no odor, but there were some who had found it highly unpleasant. At an Indian pow-wow on the Mohawk Trail in Massachusetts, one man told me,

> The smell of skunk oil depended on how the fat was tried out, how well refined it was. Many people put a drop of wintergreen oil in it to mask the smell.

Another source said, "After awhile it wouldn't smell; it would mellow out."

The first step to obtaining this wonder drug was not the rendering, however. Because of the skunk's noxious odor, I was particularly interested in how the creatures were captured to begin with. I was able to get a general picture, but wasn't totally satisfied until I ran into an old trapper from Enfield, New Hampshire. This man is a jolly, plump fellow who wears a baseball cap and still has a youthful manner about him.

> All farm boys had their favorite skunk dogs. They were a weird-looking lot of mutts, in combinations of every breed imaginable and with different types of talents. On a nice, frosty night in the fall, it was considered pretty romantic to take a young farm gal and your dog and go roaming around the fields waiting for the free-running dog to find and bay a skunk. Sometimes we would go out with one or two other couples.
>
> When a dog spotted a skunk, the fun and excitement started. Everyone would take off in a dead run. The frenzied barking of the dog and the overpowering smell of skunk made a beacon you couldn't miss.
>
> Usually we had a .22-caliber rifle with us and when the dog was in a safe spot, we'd shoot the skunk. When the hunt was over, we'd go home smelling to high heaven, laughing and joking, making comments as to who fell down or ripped the seat out of their overalls while going through a barbed-wire fence.
>
> Sometimes I'd have a skunk on a trap line. I'd walk up slowly, the skunk would face me, and I'd either shoot him or give him a sharp rap on the head with a good, solid hardwood stick. Woe to him who used a stick that broke when he rapped the skunk. The animal would whirl and give you both barrels—and they were good at hitting a running target.

After you killed a skunk on a trap line, you had about five seconds before he started spraying the countryside. To avoid this, I would some-times shoot the skunk, quickly lay down the rifle, grab the skunk by the tail with one hand and the scruff of the neck with the other. I would pull the tail up over the back, set the skunk's bottom firmly in the torn-up dirt where the trap had been, and he would spray into it.

Skunk oil was a popular treatment for rheumatism, broken bones that didn't mend properly, and colds, but in some households it had other uses. A retired nurse told me the following:

There is nothing so good as skunk oil, nothing. When I needed some of the oil, I would take a BB gun and shoot a skunk in the head. I never knew the oil to go rancid. We used it for everything. We rubbed it on the feet to keep them smooth and soft. Sometimes women even rubbed it in themselves for contraception.

Another person told me this story:

One time I lost my voice. It started out with a cold. After a while I couldn't even whisper. About five weeks, it went on. My husband said, "I'm afraid of what's going to happen to you; nothing helps. How you going to tell people what you want? You can't write." I got so scared when he said that. My girlfriend told me to come over to her father's house and have him fix me up—she said she was tired of this business.

Her father gave me a tablespoon of skunk oil and told me not to breathe when I took it so I wouldn't smell it. My friend had a sweet onion sandwich ready, and right away she had me eat a bite of it so it would kill the taste. I ate about half the sandwich, then he gave me hot tea.

You know, the next day my voice came back, and after that I never had laryngitis again.

According to one source, "If you were a weakling, your whole body would be fre-quently rubbed down with skunk oil for better muscle tone."

Instead of using skunk oil, one man actually kept a skunk in a pen. Whenever his asthma flared up, he would inhale the fumes, claiming that they would make him feel better!

SNAKE OIL

I was at a senior center in a small, rural Massachusetts town when one of the ladies whispered, "You should talk to the man who just walked in: his father was like a town doctor and a vet." The gentleman she had pointed out was short and long-waisted; he walked with a boyish stride that reminded me of characters in old-time westerns. He agreed to sit down and talk to me in a private area. As I looked into his clear blue eyes, I was mesmerized by what he told me.

Snake oil penetrates; it's highly lubricating for joints. Snake oil was from rattlesnakes. All we used was the fat lining the stomach, the outside of the stomach. It's like a lacy, white coating all over the stomach. Put it on top of a woodstove and simmer it down.

Once I put some in a little crock jar and put it in my pocket—I was going to deliver it to someone. I looked down and the pocket was all greasy; it worked its way right through the jar. Skunk oil would not do that. You have to put it in good glass.

A guy had a bad hand that was all crippled up and he came all the way from Virginia to get snake oil from me. My father used to mix snake oil with 'coon oil and give it to different people. I just threw some away he'd made in 1934; I took a whiff of it and it smelled OK, it wasn't rancid. Father put it on a cow's udder when it was caulked up—he'd rub it on to soften it up.

I used to hunt rattlesnakes in Glastonbury, Connecticut. There are quite a few in Huntington, Massachusetts. Rattlesnakes are in every state except Hawaii and Alaska; they're even found in the lower parts of Maine. They're found in certain localities, in rocky places. They live in dens. The den is always in the south-east side of a rocky hill—it's warm there. In the winter they have to go below frost level or die. They leave the den in the spring and distribute over the territory. Within two weeks, just before a heavy frost, they go back to the same den. They keep warm in the rocks. At this time of year, they're the fattest, and kind of drowsy. This is when I'd get them. You can find them lying around the den on the rocks, taking in the sun.

I used a four-foot stick with tongs. It was like a pair of pliers, it had metal hinges. Some used a loop. You grab them in back of the head. You always killed them in the head—use a stick or a rock or .22 caliber gun. They're not that hard to kill. You cut the head off and always bury it—people believed that if a kid found a head they might get poison in them.

I've sold live rattlesnakes to colleges, circuses, etc. People used the skins to make headbands, belts, even suspenders. I've done newspaper stories, been in the Hartford Courant; *but I won't let people use my name—I buck on it. I've been asked to be on the radio. I used to get calls from the police to identify them.*

I feel blessed in having been able to interview this man, because he was the only one with whom I spoke who had actually procured snake oil himself.

The greatest usage I found for snake oil was as a liniment for rheumatism. Of all the animal oils my informants discussed for this condition, it was second in popularity only to skunk oil.

In the media, I sometimes come across the phrase "snake oil" being applied to one questionable substance or another—the connotations are always derogatory. It is curious how snake oil got such a bad rap while skunk oil has no such negative reputation.

Several folks recalled that they used to buy snake oil from Indians at carnivals or fairs. Supposedly, however, there were many peddlers who claimed to be selling snake oil, when in fact, what they were hawking was something entirely different. A Native American explained this practice.

> The so-called "snake oil" that was sold in medicine shows and fairs was a mixture of different things. That, and herbal products that were sold, put Indian medicine to shame; all authenticity was taken away. Some Indians traveled in carnivals—the Indian would say he was a hundred and ten years old and used a certain product all his life. Everyone eventually came to believe that all Indian medicine was fake.

Apparently, this devious scam was already a common practice a few generations before our grandparents were born: ". . . a customer entered a store in Atchison, Kansas, in the early 1860s and asked for half a pint of rattlesnake oil. After the satisfied buyer had left with his purchase, the druggist remarked that prescriptions for rattlesnake oil, bear oil, and lard oil were all filled from the same barrel."[8]

Snake oil, the real thing, was more desirable than skunk oil. When an animal produces a toxic substance for its own defense, it is likely that some of that substance is found in other parts of the animal's body. Rattlesnake venom and skunk spray have at least one common denominator: they are both rich in sulfur. Both oils have a remarkable ability to penetrate. However, it was much easier to find skunks than rattlesnakes, and less threatening to catch them. Skunk pelts were in demand by furriers, so for many trappers, skunk oil was a side-line.

> Father used to buy snake oil at the Rutland Fair. It would cure most anything—toothache, earache; rub it on for rheumatic complaints and neuralgia. Mother rubbed it on a corn once; it penetrated right through the shoe leather.

---

[8] Laurence M. Klauber, *Rattlesnakes*, vol. 2 (Berkeley and Los Angeles: University of California Press, 1972), p. 1052.

FLANNEL

For centuries, the word *flannel* was synonymous with wool. In 1887, a reporter for the *Daily News* wrote about a new material, "a poverty-stricken article called flannelette." It was inferior because it was made out of cotton, and it became a favorite among the poor.

Flannel was used extensively in old-time medicine, especially cotton flannel; it didn't make the skin itch and it was much cheaper than wool flannel. When an oil was rubbed on the chest, throat, or aching joints, the area was often covered over with flannel; when cloth was needed for a poultice, it was the preferred material. Many wore flannel clothing in the winter to prevent illness; some wore it to aid healing. The consensus was that old-fashioned flannel kept the body heat locked in.

People often commented that "red flannel was the best." This was probably due to the alum used as a fixative in the dyeing process; alum itself is recognized for its drying properties.

Grandmothers I interviewed described how flannel was used to prevent sickness and aid healing.

> My husband had some rheumatism and his mother insisted he wear red flannel union suits in winter. I got rid of them as fast as I could after we were married.
>
> ———

> Brother had very bad back pain. He wore a red flannel band around his middle. The heat from the flannel used to cure his back.
>
> ———

> My husband didn't winter well. He was prone to respiratory infections, especially pneumonia. Each year, when the weather turned cold, I would take a large rectangle of red flannel and cut a hole in the center of it for the head. My husband would wear it all winter long next to his body; he would put his undershirt on over it. Red flannel kept the heat in the body and the cold away from you.
>
> ———

> When my child had a cold, I would take two square pieces of flannel and bake them in the oven until they turned light brown. I would fold them into quarters, then pin them to the underclothes against the body in front and in back. I would leave them on until the cold went away.
>
> ———

> When I brought home my first baby, he developed a cough. Grandmother was quite concerned and pinned a square of flannel inside of his nightshirt against the chest. When the cold went away, each day she would cut off a strip of the flannel. She didn't want the baby to have a nice warm chest one day and a cold one the next.
>
> ———

17

My mother was a beautiful seamstress. She made my father double-breasted red flannel shirts, which he wore all winter. When they wore out, Mother would save the good parts and make red flannel petticoats for me, which I wore as a first layer. The flannel slips were cut below the knees: it was believed that they would keep the legs warm and ward off rheumatism. The flannel petticoats were made very plain, but the petticoats that I wore over them were much nicer and fancier and trimmed with a lot of lace.

—

Grandma used to make us wool flannel vests. We would wear them next to our skin all winter long, from a baby until three or four years old. No sleeves, couldn't even tell you were wearing one. It would keep you warm and you wouldn't catch cold. We had a clean one for each day of the week. Grandma swore by them.

SEWAGE PHARMACOLOGY

Whenever I was interviewing someone and heard the phrase, "I hate to tell you this," or, "You're not going to believe this," I could almost be certain what was to follow. I was about to be told yet another tale of a cow-manure poultice or of the medicinal use of human urine. Other types of bodily wastes and secretions were also used, but much less often.

People have used sewage pharmacology throughout recorded history. It is still used in some parts of the world. The ancient Egyptians were more discriminating than our immediate ancestors—they used more than two dozen types of dung for healing purposes. Galen recommended using doves' dung; he devoted a treatise chapter to the substance. In the 1600s, Christian Franz Paullini, a well-respected doctor, believed that "with the aid of feces and urine, it is possible to cure, from head to foot, internally and externally, all disease, no matter how severe or poisonous it may seem to be." [9]

Several seniors had accounts for me of how various waste products were used in the past.

Dad used to say that cow dung was like penicillin. When I was seven or eight, I was running fast through the kitchen. I ran into the wood stove and the oven door fell open and burned my hand. It pulled away the skin—I can still smell it, the awful smell of burning flesh. Fresh cow manure took out the burning sensation.

—

[9] Helmuth M. Boettcher, *Wonder Drugs* (Philadelphia and New York: J.B. Lippincott Co., 1963), p. 120.

We had a large family. When diphtheria struck, Father made us horse-bun tea. He steeped it on the stove. The ones that took it lived, the ones that didn't died.

—

My brother twisted his foot and he couldn't go to school. We had an old aunt that lived with us and she went out and got a big burdock leaf and piled fresh cow manure on it. She wrapped it around the ankle and tied it on with a rag. In no time, my brother was back in school. I don't know if it was because he couldn't stand the smell, or if it really worked.

—

Mother rubbed chicken manure over my body when I couldn't break out with chicken pox. I was real sick, and I can remember lying in bed and holding my nose.

—

When we'd get poison ivy on our feet, Ma would have us walk barefoot through cowflops. I used to like the feel of it oozing between my toes.

—

I once had an excruciating toothache that I treated [externally] with a cow-manure poultice. I certainly didn't enjoy doing it, but it was better than enduring the pain.

—

In World War I, the outfit that my father-in-law was with had no gas masks. They would urinate on a hankie and put it over the face. It would keep gas away from the throat and eyes.

The following story was told by a delightful old gentleman in St. Albans, Vermont; he spoke with such excitement and enthusiasm that he kept bouncing up and down in his chair.

We used to live in Williston, Vermont, in an eighteen-room house built in 1855, the biggest house in town. A couple from Burlington used to come up and visit my folks every so often and stay a few nights. The woman was a very classy lady, a real beauty from a wealthy family. I liked her a lot and I used to cling to her. She had eczema so bad that her hands would crack right open and she would cry. The doctors didn't seem to have anything that would cure it.

An old Indian we used to call Tom-Tom worked for my folks as a farm hand. He said he knew what would cure it. That night he took her to the barn and didn't tell her what he was going to do. They waited a while; then when the cow started to take a dump, he grabbed her hands and put them right under it. I watched the whole thing—she kept trying to pull her hands back. I laughed like hell and so did her husband. The Indian bandaged her hands with the manure right in there.

You know, that actually started to heal the eczema. She noticed a difference right away. Do you realize, she came up to the barn every night to do that. You should have seen the look on her face when the cow would do that to her! Don't suppose she'd ever been shit on before!

Some seniors cited the heat that manure produces as a healing factor. And indeed, decaying cow manure generates and holds heat so well that you can dig into a pile of it at first thaw and see steam rising; and horse manure is said to be twice as "hot" as cow manure.

I have recorded the use of cow manure poultices many times in this book: the reader should keep in mind that the treatment was so ghastly that people were not likely to forget it.

- 2 -

Respiratory Problems

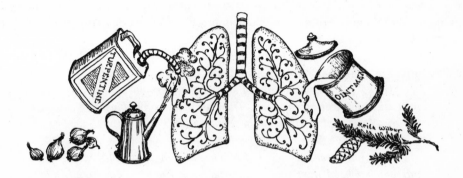

COLDS

In the past, as today, the common cold was the number-one physical complaint. I was given so many cold remedies in the course of my interviewing that if I listed them all I would have a small book.

Skunk oil. In my collection, the most popular way to treat a cold was with one of various oils; skunk oil heads the list. Some people placed a few drops of skunk oil on a teaspoon of sugar and swallowed it; others took as much as a full spoon.

> *For a cold, we'd put skunk oil and sugar on a teaspoon and down the hatch with that. It would cure a cold quicker than anything I've ever tried. It didn't smell; it had a funny, flat kind of taste.*

> —

> *On the far side of the cellarway was skunk oil, goose grease, and bear fat, to keep them cool. For a cold, Mother would give us a teaspoon of skunk oil at a time—always had to force it on us. We took it two or three times a day. Got greased with it, too.*

> —

> *When we'd get a cold we would eat some skunk oil; you can mix it in*
> *lemonade or orange juice. When the baby had a cold, I'd give him a drop*
> *of skunk oil on sugar several times a day. We had to have it in the house.*

Many chose to rub skunk oil on the chest to "make you breathe easier." It was usually warmed before it was rubbed on and then covered over with a piece of flannel. According to a little, hunched-over granny wearing a tiny black cap, "I would rub it on my front *and* back—and it didn't make me smell like attar of roses, either." Another frail grandmother told me, "I rubbed skunk oil on my chest last week when I had a cold; it's still good after all these years."

There were many variations to this treatment, such as mixing in a little camphor or a little turpentine. One man recalled using both:

> *We took skunk oil and mixed a little camphor and a little turpentine*
> *in it and rubbed it on the chest. Then we placed a brown paper bag over*
> *the area. It worked very well—the wind couldn't blow through the bag.*

> *When my sister was one year old, she had an awful cold. Mother kept*
> *putting her head next to the baby to see if she was still breathing. A*
> *friend of hers came over and rubbed my sister's chest with warm skunk*
> *oil, then sprinkled it with nutmeg and covered it over with flannel. It*
> *loosened it up.*

> *Grandma was part Indian and part French. She always kept flannel*
> *in the house. If we had a chest cold, she'd make a bag like a small pillow*
> *and slice a lot of onions and fry them. She'd drain the grease and add*
> *skunk oil while they were still hot. Then the mixture was placed in the*
> *bag and sewn up. She would put a towel on my chest and the bag over*
> *that. Boy, you wouldn't believe how that would break up the cold.*

Bear's oil. This animal fat was sometimes rubbed on the chest for a cold. An American Indian told me, "Skunk oil was the best, bear's oil was second." Someone else made the comment that "Bear's oil was good for a bad smell." There was considerable agreement on the latter point:

> *Ma had a great big bottle of bear's oil on the top shelf in the pantry.*
> *She had it mixed with quite a lot of turpentine. It smelled terrible. When-*
> *ever I had a cold, Mother would grease my chest with it, with flannel*
> *over that to hold it onto my chest . . . Father would be out hunting, and a*
> *black bear would come off and he'd shoot it. They always looked frightful-*
> *ly big to me. We didn't eat the meat or anything; he'd give it to the neigh-*
> *bors and sell the hide. Father would get the fat off the bear, Mother'd try*
> *it out [fry it] and get the tallow.*

> *When my children had chest colds, I would take some bear's grease*

and rub it on their chests and throats. My husband and his party killed two cubs. I cut the fat off the meat and rendered it until it turned to liquid and put it in a jar. We used it to break up congestion. When you cooked the fat down, boy, did it smell the house up! Had to have the doors and windows open; it smelled worse than skunk oil. We used the meat to make stew. We cooked vegetables with it to take the wild taste out of it, especially onions and celery.

Goose grease and chicken fat. These two substances were often used in the same manner as the skunk oil, both internally and externally.

An elderly couple from Brunswick, Maine, who had courageously raised fifteen children, told their story:

When one of our sons was three months old, he took on a bad cold and we thought we were going to lose him. We took a teaspoon of chicken fat and held it over the teakettle spout until it melted, and then we fed it to the baby. We did this every two and a half hours, and it pulled him out of it. It clears the phlegm and helps the bowels to move.

———

Mother had a goose every Christmas. Before she cooked the goose, she took the fat off, saved it, and tried it out. She used it on me to keep a cold off— rubbed it on my throat and chest and put a warm cloth over it.

Not everyone was convinced that such treatments were useful, though: "My mother-in-law would bring over goose grease to rub on the baby's chest. After she'd leave, I'd throw it in the garbage."

Butter. To treat colds, some ate butter. Often, a big chunk was melted in a cup of hot milk and drunk. There were variations in the way it was used to make what some called a cough syrup: warm butter and honey were mixed together; butter and rock candy were melted; some heated ginger, molasses, butter, and a little hot water. Whatever the recipe, usually a spoonful was taken three or four times a day.

Lard. Some Yankees rubbed lard on the chest; often one or more spices such as nutmeg or cinnamon would be sprinkled over the lard.

Take a piece of wool flannel—it will retain the heat. Spread warm lard on it; sprinkle it with nutmeg and smooth it into the lard so it will stay there for a while. We'd put it on the chest for one hour with a piece of sheet over it. As you wore it, the nutmeg would gradually fall off in the bed; eventually the bed would be full of it. Awful uncomfortable to have nutmeg in the bed.

Turpentine. When people used turpentine to treat colds, they most often mixed it with lard and rubbed it on the chest:

Turpentine and lard were always good for a chest cold. We used regular turpentine; we didn't get it from the drug store. It's cold when you apply it, then it gets hot; you cover it over with a piece of flannel and you leave it on overnight.

———

Melt turpentine and lard and rub on the front and back. Next day you could breathe better. That turpentine would be warm under your shirt, it would feel like it was burning.

———

We all had bad colds. Mother had pieces of flannel. She put lard and turpentine on a piece and covered my chest with it. One time—you ought to have seen my chest in the morning. It was full of big blisters with green pus. Mother broke the blisters and put Vaseline on a piece of outing flannel and placed that on my chest to heal it up.

———

Melt one pound of lard with a few chunks of camphor gum and a small quart of turpentine. Let it harden again. Rub it on the chest as an ointment. Cover it over with hot flannel.

It wasn't too long ago that Vicks VapoRub contained 4.5 percent spirits of turpentine; its label now lists spirits of turpentine as an inactive ingredient.

Turpentine was also ingested for colds, although this treatment wasn't nearly as popular as the turpentine ointments. The usual procedure was to place a few drops on a teaspoon of sugar.

Three drops of turpentine on a spoon of sugar—the greatest thing there is for a cold. My doctor said that a long time ago. Take it at night and in the morning the cold is better.

Kerosene. Some people took kerosene for their colds; again, on sugar, repeating the treatment a few times a day. One gentleman recalled that when he was in school,

The doctor told me, "You've got an awful cold. When you get home, mix a little kerosene on sugar and eat it." When I got home I told my mother, and she looked me in the eye and said, "You sure he said that?"

Camphorated oil. A number of seniors told me they had rubbed camphorated oil on the chest to break up congestion. Usually the area was covered (as in the rest of these greasy cures) with a piece of cloth.

When I was pregnant I took on a terrible cold. I rubbed camphorated oil on my neck and chest, then I took Father's long-johns and wrapped them around my neck. That broke it up.

Onions. The common onion was very popular as a main ingredient in many cold remedies. A favorite treatment was onion syrup. Some recipes call for dicing a large onion and layering it with two or three tablespoons of sugar in a bowl. Some covered the bowl so the liquid wouldn't evaporate. After the mixture sat for a few hours, it produced a watery syrup that didn't smell particularly appetizing. For a bad cold, a tablespoon of this medicine was taken every few hours—a teaspoon when the patient was a child.

In Lyndonville, Vermont, in an old inn that had been renovated for senior housing, a lady recalled a variation of this treatment that was a little more appealing.

> *I was one of fifty waitresses in an Italian restaurant in Cambridge that burnt down some time ago. It was a family restaurant, and they were the best people in the world. They always kept a jar of raw chopped onions in honey, and if any one of us started coughing they'd give us a spoonful of the mixture. If there were three of us coughing, we'd all get it from the same spoon.*

Some I spoke to had prepared the remedy in the oven.

> *Cut raw onions in big slices and place in a pie plate. Cover them with brown sugar and put them in the warm oven. The heat melts the sugar and goes through the onions and makes a syrup. When it's cool, take a teaspoon whenever you cough.*

Other people had boiled the onions along with one or two other ingredients; some form of sweetener was always used.

Some Yankees preferred an onion poultice.

> *This is a superb remedy: Fry onions in lard. Put a cloth on the chest and then apply the mixture; put another cloth on top of that. Do this and take a physic, and then if you're not better, call the doctor.*

As a cold treatment, some had placed slices of raw onions in the bottoms of their socks, usually at night. One lady told me that her father had hated onions "with a vengeance" because his mother had boiled onions and tied them in a bag around his neck to ward off colds.

Garlic. Though not nearly as popular as onions, garlic was also used to treat colds.

> *Eat raw garlic cloves to break up congestion; and it will stop you from coughing. If you can get it chewed and swallowed, you're fine. It's like eating a fireball.*

> ———

> *If you have a sinus problem or a cold, put garlic and a little chicken fat in a silk stocking and wear it around the neck. It was messy and stunk to high heaven.*

One woman told me that for a cold, she would take the skin off a clove of garlic and put the clove in a cheesecloth bag and wear it inside her bra. For prevention, some wore garlic "beads" about the neck all winter.

Mustard. Mustard was very popular in Yankee medicine. Some of my informants had taken a mustard-water bath, or soaked the feet in hot mustard water. But most used it in plasters. People believed mustard plasters were "great for everything" and that "they got warm and took the ache out of you." Although they were used for a number of conditions, they were most popular for respiratory complaints.

The plasters were usually made with common yellow mustard powder. Two or three tablespoons of flour were mixed with one tablespoon of dry mustard; a small amount of cold water would be added to make a paste that was just wet enough to spread. The mixture would be applied to a cloth, covered over with another cloth, and placed on the troubled area.

The plaster irritated the skin and increased circulation on the area where it was applied. Also, it was believed that some of the infection was drawn into the plaster.

Though effective, this old-time stand-by was potentially dangerous. If left on too long, it would blister and burn the skin. Some veterans of the treatment mentioned that they have scars from its use; many are the result of falling asleep with a plaster on. A friend told me that her father's chest was so badly scarred from a mustard plaster that it looked as though he'd suffered third-degree burns.

To avoid burning the patient, some substituted lard for the flour; some applied grease to the area before application. Others mixed in an eggwhite or milk instead of water. The plaster was supposed to be lifted every five or ten minutes to see how pink the skin was. Also, the plaster was supposed to be moved around every fifteen to twenty minutes.

Mix a little mustard powder with flour. If you use it full strength, you burn the daylights out of the skin. Mix a little water with it. Vaseline goes on the chest first in nursing procedure.

———

A mustard plaster is great for everything; it even keeps the flies off you. Pat the mixture down in a cloth, fold it up, and pin it in. I used to say to my child, "If it starts to smart, tell Mama, because that will burn you."

———

When my granddaughter was about twelve years old, I put some grease on a piece of sheet and laid that on her chest. I put a mustard plaster over that. That would break up a cold quicker than antibiotics. The next day she said, "Grandma, you're not going to put another mustard bastard on me, are you?" I looked at her and said, "What did you say? It's a plaster, not a bastard!"

———

I almost killed one of my girls with a mustard plaster because no one told me to mix anything else with it. I just used mustard and water. I left it on a nice long time. Her chest was one solid blister. It hurt so much she forgot her cold, but it cured the congestion.

It should be noted that sometimes symptoms are misleading:

> *To this day, there's nothing like a mustard plaster to loosen a cold. Use milk instead of water and it won't burn. My husband used it whenever a cold settled in his back. But then, one time it turned out to be a heart attack, and he ended up dead.*

Spirits. Various alcoholic beverages were taken in combination with other ingredients to break up a cold. Whiskey was by far the most popular, followed by brandy and wine. To the "medicinal alcohol" would be added ginger, lemon, hot water or tea, honey or sugar, or a combination. These testimonials give a fair idea of how the "toddies" and "slings" were made and what their effects were.

> *During prohibition, the doctor would write out a prescription for whiskey. We'd say we were sick just to get the whiskey. For a cold, we'd make what we called a hot toddy—we'd mix water, sugar, whiskey, and lemon, and bring it to a boil. When you drank one of those before bed, it would knock you right out.*

> ———

> *When we got a cold, we rubbed warm skunk oil on the chest, then we took a laxative. We made a hot drink of whiskey, lemon, and water and sweated it out: we called the drink a hot sling. Whiskey in our house was for medicine only.*

> ———

> *Mix and drink two shots of moonshine, one teaspoon of ginger, a tablespoon of sugar, and hot water. This will make you sweat real good, but it burns like hell going down.*

> ———

> *Boil homemade wine. After it starts to boil, put a match to it and burn out the alcohol. Add honey and lemon. Drink a small glass, as needed.*

Occasionally, a cough syrup would be made with alcohol:

> *One-half cup honey, three-fourths ounce of glycerine, one-half strained lemon, and one ounce of brandy. Mix it well and take a teaspoon as needed.*

Herbal teas and syrups. It seems that, when our elders were growing up, ginger was viewed more as a medicine than as a spice. Ginger tea was frequently taken for colds. Some took a "small teaspoon" of powdered ginger and mixed it in a cup of hot water or, occasionally, milk. A few had chopped or ground fresh ginger root and boiled it.

> *Oh, Lord, Mother used to make me hot ginger tea with vinegar and sugar in it. I'd slop over with it if I was coming down with a cold. She'd put about six quilts on the bed and make me drink that and I'd sweat something awful.*

> ———

I tried to tell my tablemates about this, but they are skeptical. Hot milk with ginger—take it after you get into bed; it makes you sweat. Really. The cold is better in the morning. Three nights in succession. I used to board college boys and I'd give it to them. It helped them out, too.

Catnip tea was also believed to be effective in fighting the common cold. This is another herb that induces perspiration—a diaphoretic. (For more on catnip, see "Nervous Complaints and Insomnia.")

Some used flaxseeds along with other ingredients to make a cough syrup. Here is a typical formula.

Take a few tablespoons of flaxseeds and boil with some water until it gets thick and gooey. Strain, but don't squeeze. Mix with equal parts of honey and lemon juice, and you have a slimy syrup. You can put alcohol in it as a preservative. You take a tablespoon at a time.

For a bad cough, some took wild-cherry bark, placed it in a pan, and covered it over with water. When it had steeped about twenty minutes, the bark was strained out and plenty of honey or sugar was mixed with it. A spoon of the syrup was taken as often as needed.

Other approaches. Some ate chicken soup, others drank hot lemonade or sage tea. Equal parts of honey and vinegar were taken, a spoonful at a time. Some chewed the underside of the slippery-elm bark. A dirty sock was worn around the neck. To stop coughing, ice water was sipped or a clove was placed in the mouth.

Other favorite remedies were mentioned:

For sinus or a cold, to clear your head, mix a quarter-teaspoon of salt in a quarter-cup of warm water and sniff it up. Repeat as you need to. It's good for a very runny nose. Some people had a special nose gadget to do it with.

—

When you first notice you're getting a cold, take a teaspoon of baking soda in a glass of warm water. It seems to ward off a cold—but you have to do it at the very first sign.

—

For a bad cough that keeps you up at night, soak a cotton cloth in ice water, wring it out, and wrap it around the neck. Then take a clean wool sock and wrap that over it to keep the chill away. This is for a nagging cough, and I swear it works.

—

I would cough so hard. Cough medicine didn't work. Mother would make me pepper tea. One teaspoon black pepper, one teaspoon sugar; pour a cup of boiling water over it and let it steep. Pepper settles to the bottom.

Take little sips as often as you need to. It would burn, but it was sure effective—I wouldn't cough all night.

—

For a cold you can't get rid of, cut up a whole lemon and boil it; strain. Mix with honey and glycerine. Take a spoonful every so often until the phlegm loosens.

This is one of the most unusual cold remedies I came across:

Inside the beaver is a certain gland, near the anus, that's about the size of a quarter. You smash it up and put it in gin and take a slug every so often for colds and congestion. We thought it contained pitch absorbed from the wood the beaver ate.

And sometimes it was not the remedy itself that was so memorable, but a particular convalescent's response to it.

The old man next door had a bad cold and was told to use a pancake poultice on his chest, because it was warm and moist. He placed a hot pancake on his chest, left it on for a while—and then the damn fool went and ate it!

CROUP

Judging by the large number of croup remedies people recalled, croup must have been quite common. When one matron related the experience she'd had with croup many decades ago, she became excited and nervous, and her hands started flying in all directions.

One night, when my son was only a few months old, I heard a strange noise. I was half-asleep, half-awake. I went to his crib and he couldn't breathe. His nostrils were sucked right in and the corners of his mouth were drawn way back because he was trying to pull in air. I was so scared. I think mothers go by instinct a lot of the time. I held him upside down by his ankles and gave him a good pound on the back. I couldn't believe how much phlegm came up—it was really thick and it felt like rubber.

Steam. Many people found that steam was an effective antidote for treating croupy children. A backwoods lady recalled the standard procedure.

When my baby had the croup, I would tell my husband that he was "mimicking a rooster" again. I would boil water in a pot, take it off the stove, and hold the child over it to breathe in the fumes. If he had it real

bad, I would place a towel or a blanket over his head to create a little tent
to keep the vapors from escaping.

An outspoken man who is confined to his wheelchair by diabetes recalled an uncommon variation of the steam treatment.

When I was four or five years old, lots of times I got croup night after
night in cold weather. I'd usually get it about one or two o'clock. I'd get
so I couldn't breathe; so I'd jump up out of bed and run downstairs as fast
as I could to my mother and father's bedroom. I'd shake their bed back
and forth to rattle it and wake them up. They had a good-sized kettle that
they kept full of water on the stove all the time. They'd put two or three
drops of turpentine in it and put it on a small stand so I could lean over it
and breathe in that steam. It cleared it up right off.

Turpentine was never used on infants. Some evidence indicates that even the fumes of turpentine can be lethal to a baby.

A further method was to steam up a bathroom well and bring the child in to breathe the moist air. Some people still use steam on croupy children: the steam cuts the mucus, making breathing easier.

Oils. Another treatment that was popular was to put a few drops of kerosene on a teaspoon of sugar and give that to the croupy child. Occasionally it was taken straight. One man commented, "We'd get more than a teaspoon of kerosene. It greased the insides. Glad nobody smoked in our house." Another man remembered treating his children with three drops of kerosene on a teaspoon of molasses: "It sounds awful, but I'm telling you, it checked it right away."

Sometimes the medical profession also used this treatment for croupy children, the dosage being as much as fifteen drops on a teaspoon of sugar. [1]

This treatment was potentially very dangerous. If kerosene accidentally went down the windpipe, it could find its way to the lining of the lungs and cause considerable damage or even death.

Another common approach was to give the child suffering from croup a teaspoon of warmed chicken fat, goose grease, butter, or skunk oil; for an infant, the dosage was a few drops. Sometimes warmed chicken fat, goose grease, skunk oil, or camphorated oil were rubbed on the child's chest and neck, and then covered with a piece of flannel.

Our family had a strong predisposition to croup. A spoonful of skunk
oil swallowed with sugar was harsh but effective. It tastes terrible.

—

Skunk oil tastes like skunk. My children had croup. When you take it,
you throw up and it brings up the phlegm; you vomit right off. My father
had to go off the reservation to get some once when I had croup real bad.

—

[1] Frank B. Scholl, Ph.G., M.D., *Library of Health* (Philadelphia: Historical Publishing Co., 1920), p. 1450.

When my daughter had the croup, I'd give her a teaspoon of hen's oil. She used to fight like a tiger because she didn't want to take it. But it was the only thing that would break it.

—

Mother would rub chicken grease on my chest. Every time she did it, I got sick and threw up. Once I threw up the phlegm, I was fine. I didn't care for chickens for a long time after that. I'd smell one and say, "Ooh, chicken grease."

—

My boy had croup, and he would get it in the middle of the night. I always used Grandma's remedy. I'd put camphorated oil on a knitted wool piece, and I'd cut up and warm onions and put them on the cloth and cover it over with another cloth. I would cover his neck and chest. The croup would go away as soon as I did that.

Silk. On a summer day, I sat outdoors in a lawn chair and chatted with a very hospitable lady from Leverett, Massachusetts.

Our family was very croupy. My brothers and I were always wearing black silk ribbons around our necks for the croup. I have pictures of me as a child with black silk ribbons on.

Another lady recalled that her son had terrible croup: "I would braid a black silk ribbon and put it on his neck, and that stopped it. People think I'm crazy when I tell them about it." Several other people mentioned using black silk, and one lady told me that she had used red.

One endearing grandmother told me that she had been married sixty-one years, and she used to run a thrift store "that the kids called a rag shop." She had learned to use an effective croup treatment that combined chicken fat and silk:

My first child was croupy. The lady that lived up the road from us had a cure for everything. She told me how to treat the baby, but it sounded so outrageous that I didn't try it for a while. Finally, out of desperation, I took some stiff, old-fashioned, cross-grained silk, and cut it into strips and braided it. Then I dipped it into chicken fat and hung it up to dry. When it stopped dripping, I wiped it with a towel to get more moisture out, then I tied it around the baby's neck.

I couldn't believe it! The baby didn't have croup again as long as he wore it. Whenever it got dirty, I replaced it with a fresh one. I went on to have six more children and I used it on all of them. With that many kids, you had to do something before you called a doctor.

Onions. Poultices of fried onions were frequently used to treat croup. Some people, though, gave their children onion syrup, which might be made with molasses instead of sugar.

The croup was so dangerous. I'd place fried onions in a bag and place it around the child's neck as warm as he could stand it. In twenty minutes, the onion plaster would check it. Kids grow out of it when they're about twelve.

—

Croup was terrifying. My mother would sit me up and put my feet in the hot oven. Then she'd make a poultice out of oatmeal, camphor oil, and onions, and place it hot on my neck and leave it on all night.

Mustard. Mustard plasters were relied on for any respiratory congestion, including croup.

I used to get croup as a child. A mustard plaster was used for that. It was put in cheesecloth or an old diaper. I hated the odor, it was too strong. My mother burned the hide right off me one time—I'm surprised I still got hair on my chest.

—

I was a bad little girl; I'd get croup until I was about fourteen. I was stuffed right up and you could hear me rattle and wheeze all over the place—I would just bark. A mustard plaster on the chest would break up the congestion and loosen the cough. If it was real bad, Mother would put a second plaster on.

Other approaches. Some wore camphor bags to treat and prevent croup. Ipecac was sometimes given to make the child vomit phlegm. A strip of rawhide was worn around the neck (one woman referred to this as her "croupy strap"). A syrup was made by boiling beet juice with sugar; a spoonful or two would be given to a croupy child.

PNEUMONIA

I was given many detailed stories on the treatment of pneumonia. When a person or family member comes close to death, the experience is likely to be etched in one's memory. Some of the tales I heard convey the extremes of fear and courage families lived with in those days when childhood mortality rates were so high.

My son had a severe case of pneumonia when he was about a year and a half old. We had him lying on a pillow on the kitchen table. My mother, my sister Viola, and I took turns sitting up with him day and night. You wouldn't know he was crying but by the look on his face. For two weeks we tried three different things, and all through his sickness we gave him a little whiskey mixed with sugar and water twice a day. The doctor had us using camphorated oil and wanted us to continue with it.

He wasn't getting any better, so my sister and I talked it over and decided to use onion poultices. We told the doctor and he said they were just a sticky mess. We fried onions in a pan and put them in a cloth bag and placed it on his chest. Whenever they got cool, we warmed a new batch. After a week of this treatment, he was in the clear.

Onions. Our forebears, when confronted with pneumonia's life-threatening symptoms, were most likely to try an onion poultice. A widely used poultice recipe called for a few onions chopped up and fried in lard or chicken fat. The combination was spread on a piece of cloth, covered with another cloth, and placed on the chest as hot as could be tolerated. Some changed the application quite frequently, and others changed it every few hours.

According to a spunky grandmother in Claremont, New Hampshire, "This treatment saved many a child with pneumonia here in town." Many people told me stories of this approach bringing about cures when other methods had failed and patients were believed to be beyond help.

When my brother was six months old and my sister was three, they both had double pneumonia. The doctor pronounced my brother dead about six o'clock at night, and said that my sister was so loaded with pneumonia there was no way she would make it through the night.

Mother was desperate. We used to raise all our own onions on the farm. Mother, Father, and I were peeling and chopping onions. Then Mom took a big pan and fried them in lard. She took a baby blanket and covered it with onions, and then she put a piece of sheet over that. She laid my sister down naked on the blanket, wrapped it around her, and pinned it in the front so she was covered with the poultice.

Mom sat up and held her in her arms all night. At first my sister could hardly breathe; but toward morning Mom could hear a little rattle. She was loosening. After a while, she coughed and coughed and spit up a lot of phlegm. About 9:00 A.M. the doctor came over and examined her: her lungs were practically clear. He said that he'd never believed in miracles until then.

Later, Mother used the same treatment on my other brothers and sisters when they had real bad congestion. Talk about antibiotics and what have you—this would never fail.

———

My mother was out at a Ladies' Aid meeting and I was left home to take care of my baby sister. We had a new pushcart and I decided to take

her for a ride; it was a lovely Sunday afternoon in October. I didn't put a
hat or a coat on the baby, though, and she developed pneumonia. My
mother and a nurse were up all night frying onions for the poultices, and
it pulled my sister out of it.

———

I had double pneumonia and the doctor said I wouldn't make it
through the night. My mother was up all night treating me with hot
onion poultices. Come the morning, I was much better, but I could taste
onions in my mouth.

I heard a number of poultice recipes that relied on the potent juices of the onions themselves, alone or in combination with substances other than the fats and oils used in frying.

My sister was three or four months old with double pneumonia. . . .
The doctor had us make a cheesecloth vest, like a two-layered undershirt.
We peeled and chopped onions, and filled the vest, front and back. Talk
about stink! It was really juicy when we first put it on. We had to leave
it on until the onions turned black—it drew the fever out. I was just nine
or ten, but I can remember because of the stink.

———

Our baby was about four months old when he developed pneumonia.
I sliced and smashed onions, then I added nutmeg. I put the mixture in a
flannel bag large enough to cover his chest. I pinned it inside his shirt to
hold it in place, and changed it every four hours because onions usually
dry out in this length of time. It drew the cold and fever out and saved
his life.

———

For pneumonia, I would take a half a dozen onions and chop them up
fine. Then I'd place them in a hot pan on the stove and add some vinegar
and flour so it would form a thick paste. I would simmer it and keep stir-
ring it for about five minutes—you shouldn't let them get mushy. You
put it in a cloth bag large enough to cover the chest, and apply it as hot
as the person can stand it. In fifteen minutes you replace it with a fresh
batch, and continue until the person perspires freely from the chest. Usu-
ally, three or four times is enough.

Whiskey. Some believed that whiskey was effective in the treatment of pneumonia, and it was best if the quality was "top-shelf." A gregarious man kept changing positions in his chair as he told the following story:

During the Depression, I was stationed at Savoy Mountain with
about two hundred other young men in the Civil Conservation Corps. I

was in charge of the dispensary. About a fourth of the camp came down with pneumonia. Everyone that had it was put in the same barracks.

Six of the boys had severe cases: they were delirious with high fevers and they couldn't be moved to a hospital. The head of the corps sent the orderly out to get some high-quality whiskey. The worst cases were given a spoonful at a time, as much as they could get into them in their delirious condition. It kicked the pneumonia out of them. In a week they were all back to normal except for one young kid that had complications with rheumatoid arthritis.

A lady in Hinsdale, New Hampshire, who had grown up with fifteen brothers and sisters recalled an occasion when both onion poultices and whiskey were used on a case of pneumonia. She told the story with such emotion that it gave me goose-bumps.

When one of my brothers was nine months old, he developed lobar pneumonia. Mother had him in a cradle in the front room by the stove: you could hear his breathing all over the house.

The doctor gave up and told Mother that the baby wouldn't be there in the morning. I was heartbroken. I said to him, "How come you're a doctor and you can't do any more?" He put the stethoscope to my brother's chest and let me listen: all I could think of was that it sounded like a roaring river. It was awful.

My mother was terribly upset and she started washing the walls. At the time, I couldn't understand that it was her way of dealing with the situation. She said, "There's going to be a funeral here tomorrow and the house must be clean."

We lived out in the country. It was so cold, and there was snow on the ground. That afternoon, I had already walked three miles coming home from school, but I had to get out of there. I bundled up and walked over to Mrs. Simpson's house.

Mrs. Simpson came home with me and said to Mother, "Whatever I do can't hurt, right?" She fried some onions in olive oil, placed them in an empty sugar bag, and put it on the baby's chest. Then she put a little sugar on a teaspoon and put three drops of whiskey on it. My brother managed to swallow it, and then he gagged and upchucked. His face was blood red. Every so often she made a fresh onion mixture and put it on his chest.

At midnight, my brother sat up in the crib and had a big smile on his face. Most of the red was gone. God, he was so cute! His hair was one mass of ringlets from perspiring so. The fever had broken, and Mrs. Simpson went home.

Mustard. In my collection, the second most popular remedy for pneumonia was the mustard plaster.

> *My husband caught a cold and it set in his lungs and turned into pneumonia. . . . He was delirious and didn't know a thing for a long time. He would say crazy things like, "Nobody could drive horses." He said he would go out to dinner with me—he got up and was going to walk right through the window. It was scary for a while. Every few hours, I put fresh mustard plasters on him, one on the front and one on the back. I used Vaseline to treat the burns from the plasters. He was sick for about three weeks.*

———

> *When I was seven I had pneumonia in one lung. I was real sick, with a high temperature; it was awful hard to breathe. Mother mixed dry mustard with flour and water to make a paste. First she would rub Vaseline on my chest so it wouldn't burn, and then she would apply it. For some reason or another she had to use red flannel to spread the poultice on. When I was critical, she did it three times—after that, a few times a day. It was real hot, and Mother kept picking it up to look at it. Every once in a while, she would say, "Lillian, you've got to cough to get the phlegm out." I got onion-juice syrup along with the treatment.*

———

> *My husband had pneumonia five times. Before I'd put a mustard plaster on his back, I would put him in hot water to open the pores. Every fifteen minutes, I'd pick up the corner of the plaster to see how pink the skin was. Don't let it get fire red.*

———

> *Mustard plasters saved my sister in 1918 when she had pneumonia and the flu at the same time. When the doctor put a mustard plaster on her chest, he said, "If that doesn't bring her out of it, nothing will."*

Oils. A number of people gave me remedies for pneumonia that consisted of simply rubbing or otherwise applying various oils to the chest.

> *My friend had pneumonia and had it bad for a long time. The doctor couldn't cure her. Finally, he plastered her chest with warm skunk oil and she came right out of it.*

———

> *Mix skunk oil with a little camphor. Cut a heart out of a brown paper bag and saturate it with the mixture. Put it on the chest and pin it to the underclothes. I pulled my baby out of pneumonia with this.*

———

One of the neighbors' twins had pneumonia with a very high, burning fever, and they couldn't afford a doctor. A tablespoon of turpentine was mixed with two tablespoons of lard and rubbed on his chest every few hours. In two days the kid was all right. When you used that treatment, it wasn't too long before you would be coughing up phlegm.

—

Doctor Higgins gave me up. A colored fellow who was no doctor at all put lard on my chest and put a hot plate on a cloth and set it over the lard. He kept changing the plates so that they would always be warm.

Other approaches. Other treatments for pneumonia were flaxseed poultices and cow-manure poultices. Those who were prone to pneumonia sometimes wore a jacket of cotton batting all winter.

Digestive Problems

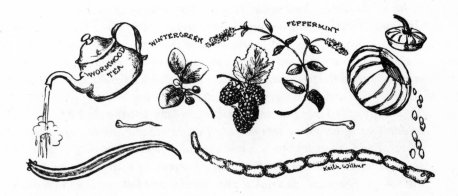

STOMACH PROBLEMS

Ginger tea. Ginger tea was a favorite preparation for dealing with stomach problems; it was used for "upset stomach" (indigestion), vomiting, gas, and "bellyache." One lady commented, "I've made more cups of ginger tea than I've got fingers and toes." A cup of boiling water was poured over a small teaspoon of powdered ginger; sometimes ginger root was chopped up and boiled to make the tea. Some added milk or a sweetener.

I spoke with a little lady who referred to herself as a "cut-up." She wore a wide smile and was neatly dressed in an old-fashioned suit garnished with jewelry. When her friend mentioned ginger tea, the following story popped into her mind:

> Old Bill lived about a mile from us. He used to go into town every Saturday night and get drunk. When he was on a good toot he always traded horses just because he liked doing it—he never had but one horse at a time. Sometimes he only had the same horse for two or three weeks. When he did trade, we all knew it right off: at two, three, or four in the morning, he'd stop in at our house and scream for my father to get out

and see the new horse he had. He'd be so drunk he'd nearly fall off the horse. Father would get up and go outdoors and put the horse in the barn and put Bill in the hay mow.

When Dad went out to do his chores, he would wake Bill up. When he was ready to leave, he'd come into the house to get his cup of ginger tea. He said it would help straighten out his stomach and sober him up enough so he could drive his horse home. That was over seventy years ago.

Baking soda. For some, the old-time baking-soda remedy was a favorite treatment for indigestion, bellyache, gas, and heartburn. The usual procedure was to mix a teaspoon or a half-teaspoon of baking soda in a small glass of water and drink the solution.

Some variations of the treatment included vinegar, which would make the solution bubble. The idea was to drink it fast while it was still bubbling.

Shortly after I was married, I took my in-laws to ten-o'clock Mass. I couldn't go in because I was so sick; I drove around and had the dry heaves. I told my mother-in-law, and she put a good inch of vinegar in a small water glass, added a little water, a teaspoon of baking soda, and a little sugar. She made me drink it as it bubbled and told me to go to bed for an hour. When I got up, it was like nothing had ever happened—I went to twelve-o'clock Mass.

Cream of tartar and baking soda. For various stomach problems, many people chose to mix a half-teaspoon of cream of tartar and a half-teaspoon of baking soda in a glass of water. Some used plain cream of tartar in a glass of water, a half to a full teaspoon; to this concoction, some added a little vinegar.

Peppermint. Peppermint tea was used to treat stomach problems and gas. It was made by steeping the leaves and the pink flowering tops in a cup of hot water until the liquid turned amber-green. Another method was to put a drop of peppermint oil in a cup of hot water; but the oil was so strong that even this small amount could be overwhelming.

Wintergreen. Some favored wintergreen tea for stomach distress. It was usually made by adding one or two drops of wintergreen oil to a cup of hot water. Occasionally, one or two drops of wintergreen oil would be placed on a teaspoon of sugar and ingested.

Some of the people I interviewed made a tea out of wintergreen leaves, and some had chewed the leaves. One source told me, "We would gather the small, new leaves, chew some, and swallow. The large leaves were OK, but they were tough to chew."

Camomile tea. Some had made a tea out of camomile and used it for stomach problems, gas, and vomiting. One lady recalled a particular occasion when, she believed, it had been effective.

My sister was very frail and she came down with a terrible cold. She couldn't keep anything down. The doctor left my mother some green

medicine which she gave to my sister after he left. But she threw it up.
Grandmother said we should try camomile tea, a little at a time, so that's
what Mother gave her. The next morning the doctor came by and said she
was much brighter. Mother didn't want to offend him, so she didn't tell
him that my sister couldn't keep the medicine down.

Ipecac. This is the powdered root of a creeping plant that comes from Central and South America. Some people purchased an ipecac preparation from the pharmacy and kept it on hand for the times that children swallowed poisonous substances or questionable items such as unfamiliar berries in the woods. It was used to make them vomit—one teaspoon was a child's dose.

Warm milk. When children drank poisonous substances, milk was sometimes given to coat the stomach.

My husband drank lye as a kid, two or three swallows—his ma
had it out because she was going to make soap. She gave him warm milk.
Butter coats the stomach too; take a few teaspoons. Butter will also keep
you from getting drunk—eat as much as you can before you go out
drinking. Keeps you sober and keeps you from getting woozy.

—

I used to work for these people, and we were out camping. About
half a cup of kerosene was left carelessly on the ground. Their ten-
month-old baby drank it. It burned his stomach pretty bad, he had a bad
time. They gave him lots of milk and cold liquids. He lived through it
and grew up.

Other approaches. Also relied on for stomach distress were catnip tea, regular tea, sassafras root-bark tea, and thoroughwort tea. For stomachache and gas, a spoonful of castor oil was sometimes taken to clean the system out; often it was mixed in a glass of orange juice. Stewed rhubarb was taken to the same end.

The following story should not be read by anyone with a squeamish disposition. It was told by a delightfully charming lady in Dixfield, Maine.

My father had terrible, terrible stomach cramps. He got them two or
three times a year; each attack would last a few days. [Possibly a stomach
ulcer.] Nobody could seem to help him. How he suffered! At times he
thought he was dying because he was in so much pain. He was given
roots and barks and different things, but finally Mother gave up and said
that she had done everything that she could.

A midwife lived a few houses down the road from us. She used to give
people advice on how to cure things. She told my mother, "If your husband
will drink it, I will make a tea and he will never have a cramp again."

The midwife went out and brought in fresh pig manure. She mixed it with cold water and strained it several times. Mother brought it to him and didn't tell him what it was. She explained that it wasn't going to taste good but if he drank it, he might never have a cramp again. I don't know how he ever got that mess down.

After he drank it, he asked what it was, and Mother proceeded to tell him—then he got nauseated! But his cramps ended, and he lived to be ninety.

CONSTIPATION

Castor oil. The castor-oil plant, native to Asia and Africa, can grow to the size of a small tree in most tropical climates. The castor bean is pressed for the oil. Many seniors could remember taking castor oil; it was the standard remedy for constipation. In many households, it was considered much more than just a laxative—it was used whenever someone got sick. If the castor oil didn't do the trick, *then* something else would be tried.

Purging has been a standard therapy throughout recorded history. People believed that, whatever the illness, the body could put more energy into healing itself when it was not clogged up. In this country, purging was still common well into this century.

The usual dose was a teaspoon for a child, a tablespoon for an adult. It was often mixed with orange juice, which helped to cut the taste; but inevitably the oil floated to the top.

Castor oil has a nauseating flavor all its own. Because of this, many seniors remembered its being used as a threat. Some mentioned that it was an excellent deterrent when a child didn't want to go to school! One lady remarked, "It was the greatest thing in the world to stop coughing—you didn't dare cough."

I grew up in a family of twelve. To make me swallow it, my mother would hold my nose. It was rotten stuff. It would make me gag, choke, and shiver. She gave it to us whenever we were sick, or a little grumpy, or a little down in the dumps and not acting the way we should be.

———

Castor oil made me deathly sick. It would run me ragged and then bind me up. We got a teaspoon no matter what we had. Ma would say, "It will clear you out and all the germs will go."

When my babies had a cold, my mother would drip castor oil on the soft spot—a laxative. She used about half a teaspoon, let it soak through, didn't rub it in. After a while, they would have a BM. And it also helped with congestion.

—

I had to lie about it whenever I gave it to one of the kids. I kept it in a bottle with no label, but they caught on shortly. One teaspoon when any-thing was wrong; it would quiet them down, help bowel movements, and bring up phlegm.

—

My father would faint away when he took castor oil. The doctor once told him he would have to take it. He explained what would happen. Dad took a tablespoon—sure enough, he went out.

Some people had a ritual of taking castor oil every week to maintain health; you could even have the pharmacist give it to you.

Every Saturday morning, especially in winter, Mother would send the three of us kids down to Kearson's drugstore with a coin, and the druggist would give us each a dose of castor oil in orange juice. It was miserable to take. I would eat crackers after I took it to keep it down. It's so thick, all I can think of is crankcase oil.

If a child swallowed a foreign object, castor oil was sometimes given to pass it out of the body. A lady in Sanford, Maine, spoke above the music of the exercise class for seniors as she recalled the following incident:

Balloons used to come with a stick attached, about one inch long. You could pull them open, let the air out, and make a lot of noise. My father was trying to read and he told me to stop it, but I had to do it one more time, and I swallowed it. The color from the balloon made me sick. I had to take a tablespoon of castor oil mixed in a cup of orange juice, and I passed it the next morning.

—

I swallowed a cent when I was small; it made cankers all the way down my esophagus. Mother gave me castor oil—she wanted that cent back. Grandmother gave me tansy tea to heal the cankers.

Senna. The native variety of senna grows up to six feet tall and is recognizable by its curved stems and yellow flowers. When the leaves or pods are ingested, it produces a strong cathartic effect. Many folks with whom I spoke had used senna to treat consti-pation, and it was occasionally used as a preventive measure or to clean one out when illness struck. In cases of chronic constipation, senna often provided the answer. It was most commonly taken in the form of a tea, one-fourth to one-half teaspoon of the leaves steeped in a cup of water. People were careful not to take too large a dose because it could cause griping.

I always had a terrible problem with my bowels. I tried this and that

*and everything, but senna was the best laxative I could find. You take
about a fourth-teaspoon with hot water and the next morning you are
sure to go.*

Some folks had made their own concoctions with senna.

*My mother-in-law had terrible constipation for about a month. She
was so sick, she couldn't eat anymore. I took some raw prunes and a little
senna leaf and ground them together, made little balls about the size of a
quarter. She took two and it did the trick. The next morning she evacuat-
ed green lumps that had been lodged in there.*

Epsom salts. Some seniors favored Epsom salts to cure constipation. One to three teaspoons were taken in a glass of warm water.

Rhubarb. Rhubarb was used as a laxative; it was taken in various ways. Most common were stewed rhubarb and rhubarb syrup. One source told me, "You would take the tip of the teaspoon of rhubarb powder, mix it with a little water, and drink." A few people mentioned that they had eaten minute quantities of rhubarb leaf, but this was a dangerous practice. The leaves contain oxalic acid, a poison that is used as a cleaning and bleaching agent.

Hot water. A cup of hot water, taken the first thing in the morning, was sometimes used to treat constipation.

Other approaches. I also heard tell of a piece of Ivory soap shaped into a suppository and placed into the rectum to cure constipation. A mixture of sulfur and molasses, half and half, was also taken—a tablespoon for an adult, a teaspoon for a child. A cup of flaxseed tea was sometimes recommended. Prunes, of course, are still taken for constipation.

DIARRHEA

Blackberry. In the days when modesty was the rule, the polite term for diarrhea was "summer complaint." A preparation made from the roots or the berries of the black-berry bush was often the chosen remedy; only one lady mentioned using blackberry leaves.

To procure blackberry roots, it was important to put on a pair of gloves, because the canes have sharp prickles. (Veteran blackberry pickers are all too aware of this!) The best time to gather the roots was in the fall, when the bushes were no longer putting their energy into producing fruit. Because the bushes often grow in dry and sandy soil, they come out of the ground without too much difficulty; but they must be pulled up slowly, because parts of the root tend to break off. One is struck by their knotted shapes and blackish-brown color. Once gathered, the roots were put aside to dry, and then they were often chopped or ground up.

When diarrhea struck, a small handful of the roots would be simmered in a few cups of water until the liquid turned a blackish-brown color. One cup would be taken; if necessary, it was followed by another a few hours later.

A small, meek woman with a slight forward bend in her posture told how the tea was useful in her childhood.

> *I had colitis when I was growing up and I still have it now—nervous bowels. Of course, when I was growing up, they didn't know what it was. My folks would boil blackberry roots and the tea would bind me right up.*

Blackberry brandy and blackberry cordials were also popular treatments; a few mentioned having taken blackberry wine.

> *Blackberry brandy used to help me out. It was just as good as paregoric. Take one good shot. If that doesn't do the trick, take another one later in the day.*

Other remedies were blackberry juice, blackberry syrup, and plain blackberries. One lady said she used to eat blackberry pie for diarrhea. A stocky woman from Manchester, Vermont, told me,

> *Take a jar of preserved blackberries from the cellar and eat one-half cupful. It would stop the diarrhea the quickest of anything. Mother didn't believe this would work, but she had been running to the bathroom for three or four days and she was getting weaker each day. I had her eat blackberries at lunch, and in the evening she told me she'd only gone to the toilet once since then.*

> *To make blackberry syrup, get the berries good and ripe. Mash them and let them make their own juice. Add a little sugar and strain if you want. Take a shotglass full. You can buy it in the store today.*

The Family Physician, published in 1849, states that the bark of the roots or the berries made into a syrup "often proves a sovereign remedy when all other remedies fail. It is a medicine much used by the Indians in dysentery; it is said that, in the Oneida tribe, five hundred were attacked with this disease in one season, and by the use of the blackberry root, all recovered, while their neighbors, the whites, fell before the disease; no doubt in consequence of taking mercury, or some of the common agents made use of." [1]

Scalded milk. Another popular treatment for diarrhea was to drink a cup of scalded milk. If the diarrhea did not subside in a few hours, another cup was taken. Often added to the milk were a few teaspoons of flour, a pinch of nutmeg, or a few good shakes of pepper.

> *For diarrhea, I would scald milk and add cinnamon or pepper. I would*

---

[1] W. Beach, M.D., *The American Practice, Condensed; or, The Family Physician* (New York: James McAlister, 1849), p. 670.

take a cup after each loose bowel movement. This works well for cats too.

———

Give scalded milk to babies in place of formula for upchucking and diarrhea in the summer. Browned flour mixed with scalded milk is also good.

Milk toast. Some of my informants had used "milk toast." (One lady referred to it as "milk soup.") Scalded milk was poured over burnt toast. Another variant of the remedy was to take burnt toast, soak it in scalded milk, strain it, and drink just the liquid. Possibly the "charcoal" absorbed impurities from the intestinal tract.

Pepper. Pepper was sometimes used to cure diarrhea. One could simply pepper food heavily, or take it in another manner.

Mother used to give a teaspoon of black pepper mixed with water, and, oh my gosh, we cried! It stopped the diarrhea. Pepper is constipating.

———

Put two teaspoons of flour in a small glass of cold water, and add lots of pepper. Mix and drink. This always worked for me.

Other approaches. Ginger tea or brandy was used to cure diarrhea. Regular tea was sometimes recommended, as was barley gruel or barley water. Castor oil would "make you go one more time." A few recalled having eaten grated apple.

Take a grated apple for anything intestinal. It had to be a glass grater, according to my mother, because the metal would somehow oxidize it. Grate it very fine. It expands in the stomach and pulls the toxins out.

PILES

Resins. The remedies I was given for piles are highly varied, and I found little consensus as to what was most popular. A scattering of people mentioned the use of resins, either plain or in mixes. (One individual mentioned turpentine, which is derived from pine pitch.) Balsam fir was used in the first remedy below.

I used this remedy on myself so I know it's true. I had terrible piles and the doctor said I must have them operated on. I was home, as miserable as all get-out. I had tried everything. I had gone from one doctor to another; they all recommended an operation. I didn't want to have the operation because my daughter's wedding was coming up.

A friend came over to drop off a wedding present. I was sitting on a hot water bottle on a chair. (With piles, when you stand up they hurt more.) He asked, "What's the trouble?" I told him and he said, "If I bring you something this afternoon, will you try it?" I said, "I'll try any-

thing." I was so miserable, no one will ever know.

He went out and got some balsam—you can find bubbles on the balsam fir tree trunk; you prick one and let it run into a little vial that will hold at least two teaspoons. He brought two vials. "This afternoon, take a teaspoon of this, skip a day, and then take the other teaspoon. Wait one month, and if you're not cured, do it again."

I detest pine smell and taste, so it was terrible to take. I ate crackers after I took it to keep it down. But that did it: thirty years later, I haven't had them since. I'm still not bothered by them. When I went to the doctor again, he said, "How are your piles?" I said, "You're going to laugh at me, but I don't think I have them anymore." He was so surprised; he said, "What have you done?" When I told him, he said that was "unreal!"

———

Rub on turpentine. Then you run around the house and scream. It burns like fire. My sister put it on her piles and screamed to her husband, "Bring me a pan of cold water!" But after that, she wasn't bothered with piles again.

———

Take pine pitch and let it firm up. Roll it into pellets, roll them in sugar, and swallow one. Do that three or four times a day, until the piles are gone.

———

Carry a chunk of camphor gum. It's good for hemorrhoids. Wrap it up and put it in your pocket. It did help me, it eased the symptoms.

———

Grandfather had piles so bad that when he died, the doctor said he must have had cancer. After he went to the bathroom, he would go to his room. There was an agate basin in there that always had clean water with creolin [a preparation of beechwood tar and resin soap] in it. There were little stacks of neatly piled sheeting, and he used to clean himself with that after every bowel movement. He had them from when he was twenty years old until he died. He would say, "At least I'm not in pain." That stuff kept them in control.

———

Put oakum in a bucket and set it on fire. Sit over it while it's smoldering. It was made from hemp with pine tar in it; they used to caulk with it.

Another source said to wrap some oakum in white material and insert it in the rectum.

Heat. Some people I interviewed had found that the application of heat brought relief. This was accomplished by using steam, taking a hot bath, or applying a hot cloth to the area.

>   *Hemorrhoids are from straining too much. My grandfather had them, and he used to sit in a large, round tub of hot water with his feet hanging out.*

Other approaches. Witch hazel was used by some seniors:

>   *Dab on witch hazel every time you go to the bathroom. It's cool and soothing. If the piles are real bad, wear a pad with witch hazel on it.*

Others had used oil-containing salves. One lady said she used to boil red clover in lard or Vaseline until the color came out, and then strain it. Below are two other formulas.

>   *Grate a carrot, mix it with lard, and insert. That will push them right back in. Do it each time it bothers you, it will give relief for quite a spell.*

>   *Boil burdock leaves in one cup of vegetable oil. Boil it until the leaves disintegrate. Strain the oil, and wash the piles with it. It's supposed to be very good medicine: it takes the soreness out and heals the piles. Apply it as often as you can.*

A couple of folks mentioned wiping themselves with mullein leaves. One good-natured fellow at a senior center in Lebanon, New Hampshire, recalled a different way his father had used mullein's curative properties.

>   *Dad had hemorrhoid trouble and this old trapper told him to go into the pasture and get some mullein leaves. You put them in a water pail, bring it to a boil, and steep them. When it cools down enough, drop your pants and sit on the pail and let the steam work up into your hemorrhoids. After it cools down more, take a cloth or cotton and bathe the hemorrhoids with it.*

>   *My dad made the mistake of doing it when it hadn't cooled down enough—the water was too hot. I thought there was a dent in the ceiling about the size of his head. He made a jump that would put a kangaroo to shame. To my knowledge, though, he never had them again after he used the treatment for a while.*

THREADWORMS AND ROUNDWORMS

Worms were much more of a problem for our grandparents' generation than they are for us today. Due to regulatory inspection of food and water, the eggs of the parasites are less likely to find their way into a person's intestinal tract.

The threadworm, also called the pinworm, used to be very common in children in this country. A lady that I visited at her cozy summer home in Halifax, Vermont, explained how to recognize infestation.

> When a kid wiggled and squirmed at night, it usually meant pinworms. A pinworm is a small, threadlike thing about half an inch long. They come out of the anus at night and you can barely see them. They're tiny, but there are usually a lot of them.

The roundworm also plagued New England communities. It has the shape of an earthworm, more or less, tapered on both ends. The color is whitish, and it can grow up to fourteen inches long. Usually when a person is infested with this parasite, there are only two or three worms. They live in the small intestine: sometimes they travel into the stomach and up the esophagus. Occasionally, they find their way into the windpipe. The symptoms are various, and include convulsions, restlessness, vomiting, diarrhea, and itching of the nose and anus.

Garlic. For both threadworms and roundworms, garlic was often the chosen remedy. It was taken in any of the following ways for one to several days, until the worms were expelled:

• A little garlic was mashed and eaten raw a few times a day.

• A few cloves of garlic were chopped up and boiled briefly in a small cup of milk; the whole concoction was ingested. This was done at least twice a day.

• Garlic was cooked in sauce or other food and some of it was taken a few times a day.

A lady dressed in a bright red suit, which nearly matched her crop of fire-red hair, recalled an uncommon variant of the garlic treatment.

> My kids were bothered by pinworms, and they used to itch their bottoms. At the full moon, the landlady would chop garlic and put it in water on the windowsill outdoors so the moon could get at it. She would leave it outside overnight, strain out the garlic, and give the kids a teaspoonful two or three times a day until the worms were gone.

There were external ways to use garlic to prevent or expel either type of worm:

• Chopped garlic was boiled in water, which was then strained. After the water cooled, it was used as an enema.

• A string of garlic was worn around the neck.

• Crushed garlic was placed on a baby's navel.

Those who suspected that their pet animals had worms often fed them a little chopped garlic every day, mixed in with their food. Many years ago, this was done to my own dog and, on one occasion, too much garlic was added to his dinner. Blue approached the bowl, took one whiff, and backed up without taking his eyes off the meal. This was one remedy that was not likely to encourage overdosing: The animal could be given only as much as it would tolerate.

Turpentine. For either type of worm, some chose to place a few drops of turpentine on a teaspoon of sugar and eat the mixture. This was done once a day, and a few people said it only needed to be done once.

After all these years, one elderly man was still irate when he recalled the time his chihuahua had worms and a friend offered to cure the dog with turpentine. Too large a dose was administered and it killed the poor animal.

Seniors told me about this treatment:

> *When kids gritted their teeth they had worms. We'd give them two drops of turpentine on sugar mixed with a little water. The next morning, all the little worms would come out.*

—

> *To prevent worms, once a month in the summer Mother would give us a few drops of turpentine on sugar. Also, every month or so she would put one drop of turpentine in a bowl of milk for the cats.*

—

> *My boy would go into convulsions. We went to a number of doctors and they didn't do any good. I suspected it was worms, so I gave him turpentine on sugar a few times; he never had another convulsion after that.*

Turpentine was never given to infants, because the treatment could be fatal to a baby.

Pumpkin seeds. To get rid of both threadworms and roundworms, pumpkin seeds were consumed in various ways:

- An ounce or two of the roasted seeds were shelled and eaten once or twice a day.
- A few ounces of the shelled seeds were simmered in a little water until tender. They were then mashed and eaten, once or twice a day.
- The shelled seeds were mashed, simmered in water, and strained out. A cup of the resulting tea was taken three times a day.

Tansy. Tansy is a plant that grows several feet high and has yellow flowers that look like buttons. Some wore a bag of dried tansy about the neck to prevent worms, and also to keep roundworms from coming up the esophagus, entering the trachea, and choking the victim.

In the rural town of Shutesbury, Massachusetts, I talked with a tall, slender old gent in a brown suit. He sat on the couch with his arm around his wife as he told me of his experience.

> *I used to get worms so bad they would come up into my mouth and nose. Whenever it happened, my mother would put dried tansy leaves in a little cloth bag and tie it around my neck. When the yarn broke, the worms would come up and I would get a nosebleed.*

A few people mentioned drinking small amounts of tansy tea to expel either type of worm. The amount consumed was small because tansy tea could be toxic.

Wormwood tea. Imported from Europe, wormwood is a plant that has firmly established itself throughout the Northeast. At one senior center, I asked a man what it looked like, and he took me outdoors and showed me a specimen. It was a rather delicate plant with lobed leaves, about a foot tall (they grow considerably larger).

Very small amounts of wormwood tea were sometimes given to expel both types of worms; it was never taken for more than a few days because it could be toxic.

> *When a child cramped up and was white around the mouth, he had worms. They could get into the throat and choke the child. Steep and drink small amounts of wormwood tea.*

———

> *Dr. Turner took me to the riverbank and showed me wormwood. "Steep the leaves and give the baby a few drops of the tea a couple of times a day." It worked. We knew that by the diapers: There would be a lot of worms in the stool. About as big as a needle, about one-fourth inch long.*

Other approaches. The following were also taken: sulfur and molasses; quassia-chip tea; kerosene on sugar; castor oil; a mild salt-and-water enema.

An unusual method was occasionally used to get rid of threadworms. A gentleman from Concord, New Hampshire, told this story:

> *Two squaws used to come to our house selling baskets. Any time my mother needed to cure anything, she would ask the squaws what to do, and they often went into the woods to gather medicine in the form of roots, leaves, and bark.*
>
> *I had two little sisters, and one of them kept squirming around and itching her bottom. One squaw looked at her and said, "Little girl has worms. Give me scissors, a large spoon and molasses." She cut off a long lock of my sister's hair and chopped it up real fine. Then she mixed it with molasses and gave her a spoonful. She told my mother to do this once a day for a few days. In a day or two the itching stopped. If I were sick, I'd rather have a squaw treat me than a doctor.*

TAPEWORM

A tapeworm can grow several feet long and cause a variety of symptoms such as high fever, nausea, vomiting, diarrhea, itching, and difficulty in breathing, chewing, and swallowing. Tapeworms are much more difficult to expel than other types of worms. I did not encounter much commentary on this subject, but the two most popular treatments appear to have been heavy dosages of pumpkin seeds and of turpentine.

Pumpkin seeds. With a twinkle in his eyes, a lovable little old grandfather recollected the pumpkin-seed remedy.

> *Don't eat anything all day: this will make the worm hungry. Then, eat something sweet—to trick the worm. Have about three-quarters of a pound of steeped pumpkin seeds ready, and eat the entire mixture right after the sweets are taken. A while later, take a laxative. (I used Epsom salts and water.) This will bring it right out.*

A similar formula was given for a child:

> *Cook half a pound of pumpkin seeds, mash them and have the child eat them. Plain is best. Wait three hours and give the child a good dose of castor oil.*

Turpentine. A lady with thinning white hair pulled back in an old-fashioned pug recalled, with horror, her tapeworm experience.

> *My sister and I would walk to the store to get hot dogs, and usually we would eat one raw on the way home. When I was nine years old, I got a tapeworm. My mother gave me some turpentine and, after a while, the worm started to come out. It's white with a black head, and all striped—an awful-looking thing. Mother had to pull it carefully so it wouldn't break. She kept pulling and pulling and pulling: it was a few yards long.*

Another approach. At the senior center in Saratoga, New York, I was given the following remedy:

> *Grandma told me this, and it's so horrible I never forgot it. When one of the boys was young, he had tapeworm. Grandma made him fast for twenty-four hours. Then she held up raw meat inside his mouth. When the head came up, they grabbed it and pulled it out.*

The above story seems to strike a note of sheer fiction; however, a similar remedy has been documented in *The Foxfire Book*. "For tapeworm, starve it. Then hold some warm milk up to your nose and sniff deeply. The tapeworm will stick his head out of your nose to get the milk. Hold the milk farther and farther away from him, thus drawing him out." [2]

---

[2] Eliot Wigginton, ed., *The Foxfire Book* (New York: Doubleday and Co., 1972), p. 247.

- 4 -

Musculoskeletal Problems

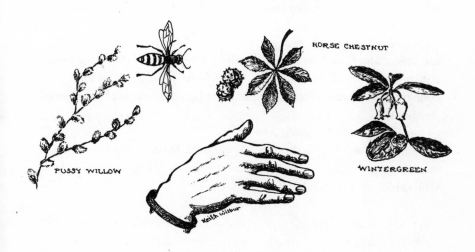

HORSE CHESTNUT

PUSSY WILLOW

WINTERGREEN

Keith Wilbur

RHEUMATISM

Although the word *arthritis* has been used in English since the sixteenth century, several people told me that it was not part of Yankee vocabulary when they were growing up. Conditions of stiffness were usually labeled "rheumatism," a catchall term that encompassed various aches and pains, and sometimes even included back problems. The incidence of rheumatism was phenomenal; those who worked outdoors during the winter months were especially prone to it.

Animal oils. Different types of animal oils were rubbed on the body to treat rheumatism; the most popular was skunk oil. The oil was well heated and massaged into the painful area as often as necessary. After rubbing in the oil, some chose to cover the area with a piece of flannel.

Skunk oil was also used for other muscular problems. One source recalled, "Father was a hunter. Any lameness—from raising a barn, or if he wrenched himself—he would rub on skunk oil." Another person remembered that when he had rheumatic fever, his mother rubbed it over the sore areas of his body.

Skunk oil could be bought at most drugstores, but that wasn't the only way to get it. I sat in an old farmhouse kitchen and enjoyed the heat of a roaring fire as I spoke with an extremely deaf, plump, and pleasant grandmother.

When I needed some of the oil, I would have my husband go out and shoot a skunk. I would skin it, clean it, and cut it into quarters; then I'd put it in a hot oven to get all the grease out. After it was about half-cooked, I'd put slices of raw potato in the bottom of the pan to clarify the oil. When we used it on rheumatism, it'd make the aching stop.

———

I would trap skunks and get from one dollar a pelt to two-fifty; the less white on it, the more I got. I would render the oil in an old pan. Father used it for bursitis and rheumatism—he swore by it. When I got done cleaning a skunk, I would smell so bad I couldn't eat until the others were done.

Other types of animal oils were used:

Father used to buy snake oil by the gallon at the drugstore. He rubbed it on for aches, pains, and rheumatism. It was nauseating to smell it. [As with skunk oil, some said it had no smell.]

———

I was partial to 'coon oil; it acted like skunk oil. I used to shoot 'coons in the fall of the year, because that's when they roam and eat. They sometimes have an inch of fat on them. You melt it down slowly on the wood stove and then bottle it.

A friend of mine was just out of high school and she got really stiff fingers and couldn't type anymore. The doctor tried different things on her but nothing worked. As a last resort, he had her soak and massage her hands in 'coon oil several times a day. It worked great and she was back at her job in no time. [I was amused when this old geezer asked me if I knew where he could find some 'coon oil: he was confined to a wheelchair and could no longer get his own.]

———

This fella was unloading a stove and it fell on his knee. It hurt his knee bad; it would tighten up. He used bear's grease so it wouldn't be laming. Didn't rub it on very often, just when it set up that way, when it tightened up.

———

I shoved my brother and he stood up quick and caught his shoulder under the door knob. It paralyzed the arm. So that was massaged with mutton tallow two or three times a day. The treatment went on for over a year. It never came back the way it should have.

Chicken fat and goose grease were also used to treat rheumatism.

Wintergreen oil. It is not surprising that certain American Indians tested the virtues of the wintergreen plant *(Kan-nah-koon-sah)* [1], for they noted that it stayed green through the four seasons. They found that a tea made out of the leaves was an excellent pain-killer, and they used it on a wide range of ailments, including rheumatism. They passed this knowledge on to the settlers and, in time, wintergreen oil was processed by steam distillation.

To treat rheumatism, many folks had rubbed wintergreen oil into the painful area as often as was necessary; some chose to put some of the oil on a flannel cloth and secure the material to the aching joint. The oil was also used to treat muscles sore from too much exercise or from the grippe, and to treat muscle spasms ("charley horse").

Some folks found that when the oil was used straight it irritated the skin, so they mixed it with animal or vegetable oil before application. People reported that this oil would create a sensation of deep heat on the skin.

Rub wintergreen oil on anything that's lame. It makes warmth on your skin. Good for sore muscles, tight joints that don't want to give right away, that have tightened up from a day's work.

———

I remember a patient that had a horrible case of rheumatoid arthritis, with swollen, angry-red joints—very painful. Every three or four hours, I'd rub on wintergreen oil.

———

My mother was crippled-up for eighteen years. She had surgery for a female problem, and couldn't walk after that. Our house reeked with win-tergreen oil. We'd give her a hot bath to open up her pores and rub on straight wintergreen oil. It didn't cure it, but it took the pain away.

In praise of this essential oil, one woman stated, "When a person had a bad case of rheumatism, wintergreen oil [rubbed into the painful area] would keep the person mentally quiet."

Turpentine. For rheumatism and related aches and pains, some reported they had rubbed on turpentine. Often it was mixed with an animal or vegetable oil or an egg to keep it from burning the skin.

Miscellaneous oils. Castor oil was rubbed on the joints; and a few mentioned using kerosene, internally and externally. Below, two people tell of unusual treatments.

[1] Marguerite R. Hickernell and Ella W. Brewer, *Adams Herbs, Their Story from Eden On* (Woodstock, Vt.: Elm Tree Press, 1947), p. 50.

Heat eel oil and rub the hot oil on. If you can stand the smell, it's all right. I put it on my knee. When I got to the store, I could smell it. It smelled up the whole store—smells like old fish. The fumes were just coming up.

———

Take a bunch of angleworms and press them. Take the oil, and throw the rest away. Rub it often on rheumatism and aches and pains, and it will cure you.

In ancient Egypt, oils were used in formulas to make the limbs "supple." The list includes such things as oil-of-worms, mouse oil, cat's oil, hippopotamus oil, crocodile oil, hog's fat, and oil-of-shadfish. [2]

The logic of the various oil treatments was very direct: where there was some degree of immobility or stiffness, the area was lubricated with oil.

Copper bracelet or wire. For many, the copper bracelet gave little or no relief. However, I did speak with a few people who swore by them.

The doctor operated on my hand for a pinched nerve. After it healed, rheumatism set in: couldn't hardly move my hand. A friend loaned me a man's copper bracelet. In two or three weeks the rheumatism went away. They say those that worked in a copper mine in Connecticut never got rheumatism.

———

I had arthritis in my knee and elbow; the elbow was red and inflamed. I couldn't pick up the arm. My husband got a piece of copper wire from the cellar and put it around my wrist. It worked in no time. I wore it for quite a while; then I took it off and wore it whenever I'd feel a problem coming on.

A friend of mine wears a copper bracelet. When it's working it will tarnish his wrist; if no arthritic symptoms are present, it will not discolor.

Another source told me, "If it turns your arm black, it does you good."

I have seen dousers at work, and even tried it myself a few times, so I cannot readily dismiss the following remedy, though it strikes a note of hocus-pocus.

This woman I know had arthritis. She was discussing it with one of the dousers in Danville, Vermont, and he suggested that she wrap copper wire on her bed springs. It actually gave her some relief.

Epsom salts and the ocean. To this day, some people still treat rheumatism and related aches and pains by throwing a couple of handfuls of Epsom salts in a tub of hot water and soaking in the solution. The medicinal use of Epsom salts can be traced to Epsom, England, where many people flocked to seek relief in the salt-laden waters.

[2] Cyril P. Bryan, *The Papyrus Ebers* (London: Garden City Press, 1930), p. 60, 64 and 65.

"Epsom salts" is the common name for magnesium sulfate, a mineral that the body is dependent on; if there is not enough of it, large amounts of calcium are excreted in the urine. Soaking in Epsom salts and hot water opens the pores and allows some of the magnesium to enter the body through osmosis.

Some of those I interviewed believed swimming in the ocean was helpful, but one woman recalled a different kind of seaside treatment:

> As a child I had inflammatory rheumatism and infantile paralysis. My uncle took me to the beach and covered me over with hot sand and had me lie like that for several hours at a time. After about three days of this treatment, I began to wiggle my toes. In time, I made a full recovery.

Horse chestnuts and potatoes. One thing I learned while interviewing senior citizens: you could never guess who knew a lot about old-time remedies. I sat with a couple in Exeter, New Hampshire. I had a gut feeling that the woman knew a considerable amount. She had long gray-black hair and a prominent nose; she looked like the storybook type who at one time would have been busy with mysterious concoctions.

She drew a blank.

The gentleman who sat next to her had not been made less handsome by the years. He wore khaki clothes and sat there quietly, taking it all in. Then he started to speak:

> Dad used to have rheumatism—that's what we called it in those days—so he carried a horse chestnut in his pocket all his life. It worked for him and it works for me.
>
> About twenty years ago, I thought I was getting arthritis because I was getting stiff, so I started carrying two horse chestnuts in my pants pocket. I still carry them. [He took one out and put it on the table.] As long as the shell is not cracked or broken, it will work. When I start to stiffen up, I pull them out and check for cracks: if they have any, I throw them away and replace them with new ones.
>
> Ten years ago, a friend of mine up in Kittery was walking with a cane—and not too far, either. He'd reached a point where he would try anything. I told him what to do, and now he's walking better than me. I've given horse chestnuts to five other people with arthritis, and they're all better than they were.
>
> I think this is an old Indian remedy. Most people laugh at me when I tell them about it, and I can't say that I blame them. Maybe it's all in my mind. I guess if you believe in something, then it works.

It is said that Dr. Oliver Wendell Holmes faithfully carried a horse chestnut in one pocket of his greatcoat and a potato in the other to protect himself from rheumatism. [3]

---

[3] M.F.K. Fisher, *A Cordiall Water* (Boston and Toronto: Little, Brown, and Co., 1961), p. 163.

A few people mentioned carrying a potato in the pocket to cure or prevent rheumatism. When the potato shriveled, it was replaced by a new one. One man mentioned putting a small, raw potato in his stocking and wearing it during the day.

Stings. Honeybee stings sometimes cured rheumatism.

A journey over the Mohawk Trail (which affords a splendid view of the Berkshires) brought me to Williamstown, Massachusetts. In the local nursing home, I chatted with a lame resident who sat with a homemade patchwork quilt on her lap:

> *My father raised bees for honey. He had some difficulty getting around because he was badly crippled with rheumatism. When any of the neighbors had a hive in a tree, they would call him over to get rid of the bees. One time he was doing this and a branch on the tree caught his veil and his big hat came off. The bees went down his shirt—they were all over him.*

> *His friend threw him in a water trough and then slapped mud on the bites and gave him lots of whiskey to drink. The neighbor claimed that he would be cured of his rheumatism and that he would never get it again. Most of it did go away, and it didn't come back for about twenty years.*

In Caribou, Maine, I spoke with a man who had been named after a minstrel singer "who could really sing and dance." His story indicates that hornet stings may be equally effective.

> *My friend had rheumatism so bad he could hardly use his hands anymore. He was picking fresh raspberries, and he ran into a hornets' nest; it was in a bush a few feet off the ground. He was stung several times. After that, his hands were so good, he got back to playing the piano.*

In Middlebury, Vermont, a thin, articulate man told me the following story:

> *Through the years, many old-time beekeepers told me about this. I would say to them, "You're crazy, you're nuts." In 1934, I had rheumatic fever. The excruciating pain migrated to every part of my body and I never slept for two weeks. It improved, except for the pain in my knees. One day, just to see if it would work, I placed a stinger on the trigger point of each knee. [You press over the entire arthritic area, and when you feel a sharp pain, that is a "trigger point."] The next morning I woke up and noticed that something was different—then I realized that my knees didn't hurt anymore.*

Barks. Occasionally, willow-bark tea was used on rheumatism. A Rhode Island medicine man with long, graying hair pulled back in a ponytail gave me the following information:

> *The best pain-killer is from the pussywillow: you scrape the bark, boil it, and drink the tea. When anyone comes to me with arthritis, I recommend the sweat lodge and willow tea.*

Trappers who lived outside all the time used to put a teaspoon of willow bark in the coffeepot to ward off rheumatism. It was called black medicine.

A few people told me they had successfully used slippery elm to cure their rheumatism.

My mother's knees were so bad that she could barely get around. A friend of ours, Corn Planter, took elm bark and boiled it down in water. He brought a gallon of it over to my mother's house and told her to take one half cup of the liquid three times a day. Before one fourth of it was gone, she was better; and by the time she finished the jug, she was completely cured.

Other approaches. Equal parts of honey and vinegar were mixed together; one or two tablespoons were stirred into hot or cold water and taken daily. Hot packs were applied. A strip of silk was worn on the wrist or ankle. And if an adrenaline rush can cure rheumatism, here's one for you: "Take a black widow spider and have it crawl on you every so often."

SPRAINS

Epsom salts. The most popular way to treat a sprain involved the use of Epsom salts. Often, a cup or two would be added to a basin of hot water and the injured part soaked in it. Some chose to dunk a rag in a strong, hot solution, wring it out, and apply it; when the application cooled, it was changed, and the process was repeated until the pain was relieved and the swelling reduced.

A large-boned Vermont farm gal explained how she had treated a knee sprain.

We were living on this old farm way up in Landgrove. One night my husband went out to the barn to do his chores and slipped on ice and hurt his knee. Next morning, the knee was all swollen and he could hardly move—he couldn't get up. We were afraid it would go into rheumatism.

After breakfast, we heated about a quart of water with a cup of Epsom salts, took a piece of cloth, put it in an old potato ricer, and dunked it in the solution. Wrung the water out with the ricer, picked the material up by the corners, and put it on his knee.

He screamed—he thought we were cooking his knee. Just the minute it started to cool, we'd put a hot one right on. In the evening, he was able to do his chores again. When he got done, we started the treatment again, and kept it up through the second day. Never had no more trouble with that knee.

Other salts. Some preferred salt pork or corned beef brine. It was used in the same manner as the Epsom salts, soaking the area directly in the hot solution, or dipping and soaking a cloth and wrapping it around the sprain.

A few people gave me remedies that called for table salt. An eggwhite might be mixed with salt, made into a paste, and applied; or the remedy could be more complex, such as the following:

> Two tablespoons of salt, two tablespoons of camphorated oil, three
> tablespoons of ammonia, and a pint of water; mix together. Soak cotton in
> it and bind it on the sprain. Leave it on.

A lady from Springfield, Vermont, told me she had put salt herring on her sprained ankle and it took away the swelling.

Turpentine. Sometimes turpentine was rubbed on a sprain. A man from Tolland, Massachusetts, had used a different method: "For sprains or leg cramps, I would dip a string in turpentine and tie it around the ankle. It was good for the whole leg."

One old Yankee was inclined to ramble on, getting sidetracked so often I had to keep drawing him back to the topic at hand:

> Use turpentine on you and you get results. The health nurse won't
> let me use it anymore. Use it on a sprained leg or arm. On the feet, it's
> the best thing in the world to take soreness out and heal things. Good for
> a sore on the foot—not open—or if you bumped yourself.
>
> I used it on the horses if the collar hurt their shoulders. Apply it
> straight; but don't rub too hard, though, because it irritates and is too
> strong.

Wintergreen oil. This substance was applied straight or in combination with other things.

Animal oils. There were those who were partial to rubbing animal oils on sprains. The list includes skunk oil, bear oil, woodchuck oil, snake oil, goose fat, and chicken fat.

> My son used to play baseball. When he pulled muscles, I would take
> skunk oil, add a little wintergreen, and rub it into his arm. It worked so
> well that the coach wanted to know what it was.

Vinegar. Some had rubbed in vinegar, either plain or in combination with other things. The lady who told the following story had a touch of indignation in her voice, the success of the cure notwithstanding:

> My husband was a vet. I pulled my ankle. He tore up an old sheet
> and dunked it in vinegar and bandaged it on. It took the inflammation
> out. He treated me just the way he would a horse.

Other approaches. Other products that were rubbed on sprains included kerosene and witch hazel. Sometimes hot packs were applied. Plantain leaves were bruised and bandaged on.

A few seniors I interviewed remembered wrapping an eel skin over a sprain. At the senior center in Gardner, Massachusetts, I talked with a man who used to procure medicinal plants for the government.

I had an awful pain right here [pointing to the top of his wrist] and a bump in there about the size of a pea. I would go to get up, put my hand on the arm of the chair, and I wouldn't be able to get up. The doctor thought I had a broken wrist and took X-rays, but nothing showed up.

A man I knew, who was about seventy years old, said, "You come over to the house and I'll fix it up and I guarantee it won't hurt anymore." He caught and killed an eel. He cut it all around the neck, sliced it down the back an inch or two, and pulled the skin off. He wrapped it on my wrist and put gauze over it to keep it in place. It smelled like fish—there's oil in the skin even when it's dry. Left it on for five days and never had another problem. It took the lump away.

BROKEN BONES

In the generations preceding ours, methods for dealing with broken bones were similar to current treatment. If a bone broke and snapped out of place, the first consideration was to pull the sections back into place.

I was alone in the woods hunting. I was on a cliff when I slipped on ice. My leg broke; it was dislocated. I put my leg in the crotch of a tree and pulled on it until it went back into place. The pain was unbearable—I thought I'd pass out, but after I did it, I was able to make it back home.

Splints. The second consideration was to protect the injured limb. For self-treated people, this usually meant a splint. When preparing the splint, the limb was usually well padded, and then two or three pieces of board or sticks were wrapped on with rags.

A few people recalled rolling newspapers tightly to serve as a splint. One man claimed, "I've even seen them use two branches wrapped on with a shirt." A woman recalled she'd had considerable difficulty putting a splint on her pig's broken leg!

Casts. A few people told me they had used plaster of paris to make casts. The substance is a fine white powder consisting mostly of calcium sulphate, which comes from gypsum. When the powder is mixed with water, it forms a paste that dries into a hard cement.

One man was delighted to tell one of his favorite stories about a troublesome cast put on in the doctor's office.

In 1927, when I was ten years old, I fell in a cellar hole and broke my shoulder. I had a cast on the shoulder and all around it. When it came time to take it off, the doctor marked it with a wheel and said, "Your father can cut this tonight when you get home." He said to use vinegar in the cracks to dissolve the plaster.

Father couldn't get it off—used screwdrivers and everything else. The doctor finally got it off the next day. It was made of Portland cement: the nurse had got the wrong stuff.

About twenty years later, the doctor said, "I'll never forget that cast."

Starch was occasionally used to protect the injured limb. "It used to come in a blue box with a picture of an Indian maiden on the front." You could make the starch as thick as you wanted; I have a vague recollection myself of clothes starched so stiffly they could stand up on their own.

For a broken bone, soak it in hot water; first test the water with your elbow, because the bone is very sensitive. Rub on skunk oil. Make a cast: starch a piece of cloth and put it on wet.

You can tell if the bone's getting better by the way a person squirms when you dress him—if it hurts awful, he's not doing well. In four or five days, take the cast off and wash the area. Rub on skunk oil and put on a new cast.

People were sometimes creative in their efforts to protect a broken bone. A straightforward grandmother who spoke in a monologue seemed oblivious to the chatter all around her as she recalled when her mother fractured an elbow in 1905.

Father took part of a stove pipe and cut it in half down the middle. He bent it to fit the arm. Then he padded it real good on the inside and slipped it over Mother's arm and wrapped strips of sheeting over it to hold it on. When it healed, skunk oil limbered it up—still had an aroma to it, too.

A lady in her late nineties, who had grown up in a rural mountain town, kept her rocking chair going as she told the following story.

My father's fingers were crushed real bad by farm machinery, and he was going to cut them off. My mother bandaged his hand and then shellacked the bandage, and his fingers were saved.

Animal oils. Many accounts mentioned rubbing skunk oil on a broken bone before applying a splint or a cast. More important, when a bone didn't mend properly, repeated treatments with warm skunk oil reportedly went a long way toward returning the bone to normal. To effect results, this treatment had to be continued for several months, and sometimes for over a year.

My mother fell and shattered her elbow so that the arm was all contorted. I shot some skunks and hung them up. I took the fat and put it in a double boiler until it melted; then I bottled it. I brought two quarts to my mother, with instructions to heat it until it was very warm, then massage it in and cover it over with flannel. She was to do this at least two times a day.

This straightened the arm in a year and a half. The doctor couldn't believe that the arm straightened, and asked her how she had done it.

———

My friend, Leon Moon, accidentally got shot in the shoulder. The wound left his arm in such a state that he couldn't raise it from the side—couldn't move the arm at all. I'd stick a bottle of skunk oil in a pan of warm water and heat it, and rub it on his arm three or four times a day. In time, he was able to raise his arm, though it never became perfect.

———

I was cutting wood with a double-bladed axe, and my hand was too close. When I came back with the axe, I cut my thumb off, and cut my index finger past the bone. The doctor in town wanted to cut my finger off, but I wouldn't let him. When it healed, the finger was crossed over to my little finger, raised in the air, and I couldn't bend it.

I went to see an old doctor in St. Johnsbury and had him look at it. He told me to take skunk oil and rub it on a few times a day, and said that one day I'd be able to bend it; and I did. It took several months of treatment. There was no way I could move that finger until I treated it with skunk oil.

In Johnstown, New York, I spoke with a man who had tried bear's oil.

When I cut that finger off, it was sewed back on, and it's always been crooked. After it healed up, I rubbed bear's oil on it to try to straighten it out, but it didn't work. It was supposed to lubricate the cords.

I was in the little town of Wellfleet on Cape Cod, where I hoped to interview a spry little old man whose face was intensely wrinkled. He was in a great rush, but he did manage to pacify me with one remedy. He said it was an old Indian cure for broken bones and sprains. He requested that his name not be used, "because I don't want my phone ringing off the hook."

Take a half a pint of night crawlers and a half pint of heavy cream. Bring it to a boil, simmer it for ten minutes. Let it cool. Skim off the top. Use the stuff you skimmed off for broken bones; rub it on a few times a day. I had a friend that broke some fingers and he couldn't move them. After two months of this treatment, his fingers were fine.

The Pocumtuc Housewife, written in 1805 by the ladies of Old Deerfield, Massachusetts, states, "An ointment made of ground worms simmered in lard, and rubbed on with the hand, is excellent when sinews are drawn up."

Another approach. Comfrey tea was drunk to help bones knit; one lady mentioned a comfrey poultice.

- 5 -

Neurological Problems

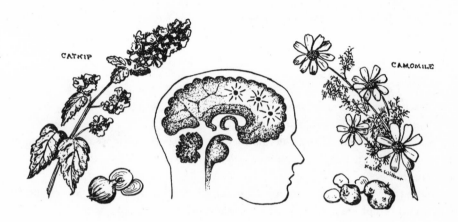

NERVOUS COMPLAINTS AND INSOMNIA

I have grouped nervous complaints and insomnia together because the two problems are closely related and because both conditions were usually treated with either catnip or camomile tea. In general, these two herbs appear to be similar in action.

Catnip tea. Catnip tea was the medicinal beverage most frequently given to babies and children. Some older folks felt that it was much more effective to give this brew to unruly children than to keep them in line with threats or punishment. It was also used to put children and babies to sleep.

I don't mean to give the impression that catnip tea was reserved exclusively for children; adults also drank it, but less commonly. A few people told me that they had used catnip tea "to cure everything." Some adults had taken the beverage freely for nervous disorders, including nervous breakdown. One informant told me, "Catnip tea is good for anyone that's nervous. It will either make you active or simmer you down, depending on what you need." A man explained it was most helpful when he "hit rock bottom" and decided to "dry out": it soothed his nerves and cut down on the DTs.

Although the following anecdotes are quite similar, they show how people found this herb helpful.

> *Catnip tea worked wonderful to calm the baby down, especially when he was teething. Usually it put him to sleep. When he got older, I gave it to him when he was down in the dumps, despondent, or didn't feel good.*

> —

> *My mother would give me catnip tea and tell me it was to make me good-natured. It would calm you down if you were disturbed or out of sorts.*

> —

> *I gave my kids catnip tea when they yelled a lot and cried a lot, and I gave them a cup just about every night to make them sleep. My husband and I drank it too—it had a tonic effect.*

One lady remembered the time that her neighbor had a six-and-a-half-pound baby that couldn't tolerate milk, so the infant was given catnip tea. "It's calming and good for the stomach."

Catnip tea was made by steeping a tablespoon or more of the dried leaves and flowers in a cup of hot water. A Native American told me, "Catnip has a lot of medicinal value, but it's not very strong medicine."

Catnip is a member of the mint family; it's a relative of spearmint and peppermint, and has similar properties. These "relatives" are herbs we use on a daily basis as flavoring agents in toothpaste and sweets.

Camomile tea. Many folks who were plagued by insomnia had a standard, tried-and-true remedy to induce sleep—they simply took a hot cup of camomile tea before retiring at night. It was also useful for soothing frayed nerves when problems mounted and life seemed to get out of control.

The tea was made by pouring a cup of hot water over a tablespoon or more of the yellow blossoms and letting it steep until the color came out. Camomile tea was most frequently taken by adults, but it was given to children and infants as well. A baby's dose was one or two teaspoons.

People believed that, like catnip, "camomile was good for everything," and they gave me enough miscellaneous uses to show they meant it. Part of an old rhyme indicates that it even works to heal other plants.

> *Therapeutic camomile*
> *Placed near a plant that's sick*
> *Brings it back to health again;*
> *Propinquity does the trick* [1]

---

[1] Marguerite R. Hickernell and Ella W. Brewer, *Adams Herbs, Their Story from Eden On* (Woodstock, Vt.: Elm Tree Press, 1947), p. 41.

HEADACHES

Potato. The most popular headache remedy involved taking a raw potato and cutting it into thick slices. The slices were wrapped in a piece of material which was then tied to the forehead as a headband. Several people told me that when the slices turned black, the headache would be gone.

Three seniors contributed variations of this remedy.

I remember Mother's cure for a migraine headache—she had terrific ones. She would slice a big potato in half and place the raw surface over the site of the pain. She'd also put a rolled-up towel around her neck and twist it as tight as she could. She always claimed it worked.

―

Slice a potato and put pepper on the pieces. Wrap and fold in a hand towel and tie it on the forehead with the peppered side against the head. Once I left it on overnight and it burned something awful.

―

For a headache with fever, peel a potato and then slice it about three-sixteenths of an inch thick. Put the slices in a bowl and cover them over with white vinegar. Let them stand ten to fifteen minutes. Put the potatoes flat in a towel and make a headband, tie it in the back, and go to bed. The vinegar would draw the fever out.

Cold water and ice. Many seniors simply dunked a cloth in cold water, wrung it out, and secured it to the forehead; when ice was available, it was wrapped in the cloth.

For a headache, put a cold cloth on the forehead and a hot-water bottle at the feet. Seems like I never saw Grandmother without a rag around her head. When the ice man went by, she'd steal a piece of ice and wrap that in a towel.

Vinegar. Some told me they had soaked a cloth in vinegar and secured it to the head. A few people mentioned saturating a piece of brown paper bag with vinegar and tying it on the forehead. One lady told me she used to put sauerkraut on the temples; another had soaked burdock leaves in vinegar for half an hour and then applied them.

Camphorated oil. This was sometimes rubbed on the temples or placed in a cloth which was secured to the head.

Other approaches. Slices of raw onion were secured to the forehead. A cloth soaked in rubbing alcohol was tied around the head. Witch hazel was rubbed on the temples or placed on a cloth which was secured to the forehead. Regular tea and willow-bark tea were sometimes taken.

This was one woman's formula: "For a terrible headache, pick up a knife and make a cross in front of your face with it, then throw the knife on the floor."

- 6 -

Eye, Ear, Nose, Mouth, and Throat

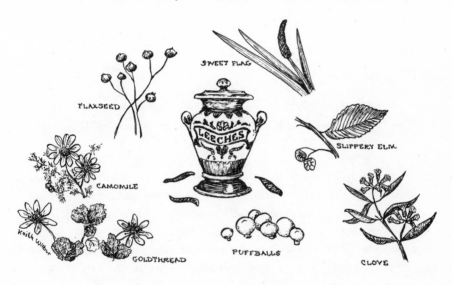

EYE PROBLEMS

Milk and cream. Many of our grandparents used milk or cream from the family cow to treat their eye problems. People spoke of using them on tired or sore eyes, pinkeye, styes, granulated eyelids, itch, ulcers, infection, a particle in the eye, and burning eyes. (The ancient Egyptians included milk in many of their eye treatment formulas. It was included in remedies for such things as cataract, leucoma, blood in the eyes, and film in the eyes, and in treatments for improved eyesight.[1]) A number of senior citizens used it as a general eyewash and said it had a soothing and drawing effect. The milk or cream was often warmed before a few drops were placed in the troubled eye and left to set. A handful of people recalled using human breast milk and said that it worked especially well.

A short, wiry man from Corinna, Maine, described the time his eyes had become infected.

---

[1] Cyril P. Bryan, *The Papyrus Ebers* (London: Garden City Press, 1930), pp. 95–99

I used to work in a lumber mill, and one day I was jumping log to log to cross a thirty- to forty-foot pond. I fell in and my eyes turned red; when I woke the next morning both eyes were sealed tight. I probably got the infection from the oily film on the water, created by the softwoods.

I sponged my eyes off with milk when I woke each morning, and several times a day I took an eyedropper and placed four or five drops of milk in each eye. In less than a week they were all cleared up.

———

Milk drops in the eye for eye ache, right from the cow. There was one special cow we used, I don't know why. Do it three times a day. It's very soothing.

———

If you had something in your eye—metal, dirt, et cetera—a few drops of warm, raw milk will flush it out just like a flaxseed. Later, wipe with a clean cloth and the particle will be in the corner of the eye.

———

Breast milk is the best. When my brother was a small baby he had some eye trouble: scaly crusts. Mother was nursing and she squeezed out some milk and washed his eyes with it a couple times a day.

Tea. Another method of treating eye problems was to apply to the eyelid wet tea leaves, a used tea bag, or a cloth that had been soaked in tea. This treatment was used on such diverse conditions as runny eyes, conjunctivitis, particles in the eye, swollen eyes, sticky eyelids, and eyes that were red from a hangover. The application was reported to be most effective when left on the eyes overnight.

A tiny, spry lady tried to keep her overly friendly mammoth dog, Rain, off me as she explained how she had found tea bags to be advantageous in her courting days.

When my friends and I were getting ready to go out on a date, part of the ritual was to place cold, used tea bags over our eyes for about twenty minutes. It would take all the puffiness out and make the eyes bright and shiny.

———

When my son was about sixteen, he was outdoors in the evening welding with no protective glasses on. It blinded him. He couldn't see at all. I kept soaking gauze in hot tea, and placed it over his eyes as hot as he could stand it. I was up all night doing it over and over. The next morning most of his vision had returned. When I was able to get him to a doctor, he told me that the tea may have saved his sight.

———

I had a foster boy and he was subject to styes, real bad ones. He would wet a tea bag and tie it around his head with a bandage—he looked like a pirate. He would wet it every time it dried out. In a couple of days the stye would be gone.

———

They used to call me `the Nurse' on my street. I've been with a lot of people in the nursing home while they were dying. . . .

For sore, sticky eyes, you make a good, strong tea, let it cool, and wash your eyes with it. My little granddaughter had a very sore eye—it would run, and got white, crusty stuff on it. It was swollen and she couldn't open it way out.

I made this strong tea and let it cool. I took a face cloth and dunked it in the tea and put it on the eye and had her hold it there for ten minutes—you keep dipping it in and out of the tea. At first she didn't want to do it. I told her I was giving her eye a drink of tea. It made her eye feel good afterwards and she started asking for it. We did it three times a day, and it took two days to clear up.

Flaxseed. A man who had worked around coal engines all his life described a method that was sometimes used to remove a particle from the eye.

Occasionally, one of the men would get a cinder in the eye and, to get it out, they would place a flaxseed in the affected eye. It would pull the cinder out and move it to the corner of the eye where it could be easily removed.

People told me that the seed works itself right around and comes back to the corner.

Other approaches. The eyes were also washed with a weak solution of boric acid and water, or bathed with a mild witch-hazel-and-water solution. Sometimes a stye was rubbed with a gold ring several times a day. Raw beef was sometimes placed over a black eye. A few people recalled licking objects out of someone's eye. Warm camomile tea was used as an eyewash and compress; one woman told of a variation.

For an abscess or any eye problem, take the dried flowers of camomile, place in a small cloth bag, and steep in a little water. Place it on the eye as hot as you can stand it, and press as hard as you can bear. Do this several times a day. This will draw out the pus and heal the infection overnight.

For a black eye, a few had used leeches "to pull out bad blood" trapped under the skin. This practice was an offshoot of the earlier days of the barber-surgeons, when bleeding was highly recommended in many illnesses. (In fact, when George Washington came down with the flu, his doctors took so much blood that within twenty-four hours he was dead.)

I sat at a table with a group of women at a senior center in Laconia, New Hampshire. When a lady told this story, she had her peers laughing.

> When my brother came home from the war, he was living it up and getting into mischief. He was in a barroom brawl and got two good black eyes. The next day he was supposed to stand up at his best friend's wedding.
>
> It was nighttime and the drugstores were all closed. [Leeches could be purchased in drugstores.] His friends went to a nearby pond with flashlights and caught bloodsuckers around the banks. When they got back, they put a bloodsucker under each eye. They would fill up with blood and then fall off. As soon as one would fall, they'd put another one on.
>
> The next morning, all he had was red spots around his eyes: the black was gone. You couldn't tell he'd been in a fight. He just looked like he'd been on a good toot.

I am told that Rattlesnake Pete from Rochester, New York, has passed on; it would appear that, to some, he has become a legend.

> Rattlesnake Pete in Rochester took leeches from Conesus Lake—it was loaded with them. He took them to his shop. He'd put leeches on a black eye; an hour later the black would be gone.

EARACHE

All of the earache treatments in my collection involve the application of a warm substance. A druggist with whom I spoke told me that once when his child had a bad earache, they bundled him up in a hat and coat and started for the hospital; by the time they got there, the child was sound asleep. The pharmacist attributed this to the heat from the hat.

Oils. Many of us can remember warm oil treatments for earaches: the head would be tipped to the side and a few drops of oil would be placed in the ear canal. (Hot oil was *never* used.) The favorite mentioned was "sweet oil"—olive oil. Also used were skunk oil and butter. The oil wasn't heated up directly; the spoon was warmed by placing it in hot water, or on the stove, or by heating it with a match, and then the oil was placed in the spoon. After the oil was in the ear, the canal was plugged with cotton batting. The treatment was repeated two or three times a day until relief was obtained.

The same pharmacist said that this treatment could cause the ear drum to perforate. Although it seems that it would have been safer to place a warmed medication on a piece of cotton and place the cotton in the ear, tradition endorsed both approaches.

None of the stories told are as dramatic as the following, which came from a lady from East Longmeadow, Massachusetts.

One night, when my daughter was five or six years old, she woke up screaming—she had a bad earache. I put a heating pad and different things on it. Nothing happened.

I remembered my grandmother saying that sweet oil was good for an earache. I heated some sweet oil in an egg poacher, and then put it in an eyedropper. I placed quite a few drops in the ear canal. In about half an hour she went to sleep. When she woke up the following morning, the pillow was covered with a green and yellow guck. It was the thickest stuff—you wouldn't believe the amount that could come out of an ear. I was scared to death; I thought I'd cleared her whole head out.

It was Sunday and I couldn't get the doctor, so I put some mineral oil on a cloth and wiped around the ear to clean it up. I didn't dare put anything else in the ear. But the ear didn't ache anymore. Apparently, it had been abscessed and the oil had broken the abscess.

Some chose camphorated oil to deal with earaches. This oil was not introduced directly into the ear in any of the accounts I heard, but was warmed and drizzled on cotton.

When I was four years old, I was jumping on the bed with a pencil in my mouth. I fell off the bed and the pencil punctured my ear—it pierced it from the inside. My mother placed camphorated oil on cotton and put it in the ear canal. It took the pain away. Every time the ear hurt, she would do this.

Smoke. A common method of treating an earache was to have someone blow a mouthful of pipe, cigarette, or cigar smoke directly into the ear canal. The ear would then immediately be blocked with a piece of cotton batting. Some repeated the process every five or ten minutes, others waited up to two hours; it depended on the severity of the earache. One lady told me that whenever an earache flared up, she couldn't wait for her father to get home from work to administer the treatment.

A woman recalled a remedy that was a little more complex.

When I'd get an earache, Father would put plantain leaves in the oven and heat them. First, he'd blow pipe smoke in the ear; then he'd place a hot leaf over there, and a piece of flannel went over the whole thing. He kept doing it over and over, until the ache was gone.

Urine. For those who got no relief from the above treatments, fresh urine placed in the ear sometimes provided the answer. One woman who had believed this to be an effective remedy said, "The urine should be from a child under ten. The doctor used to say, 'Use that and never have mastoids.'"

An Indian woman had me urinate in a pot. She told me to lie on my side and she filled my ear with the urine. The earache went away, but I cried all day because of the humiliation of having urine in my ear. [Another lady told me that her grandmother had done this to her and she'd never forgiven her for it.]

—

When one of my babies would get an earache, I'd soak cotton in their urine and squeeze two or three drops in the ear. Grandma said it was the salt in the urine that killed the pain.

—

I would get terrible earaches and cry from the pain. I tried warm butter and different things and the doctor gave me drops that didn't do any good. Finally, our landlord, who lived next door to us, made me urinate in a little glass, and then lie on my side. He put a few drops of the urine in my ear, and then plugged it with gauze. In twenty minutes the ache was gone. The urine must be fresh and warm.

Onion. Some people preferred an onion treatment. The onion would be baked or boiled and placed over the ear as a poultice. Another method was to bake or boil an onion, pull the heart out, and place it gently in the ear canal.

Salt pack. A salt pack was sometimes made. The salt was heated on top of the stove or in the oven, placed in a small cloth bag, and laid against the ear. When the salt lost its heat the treatment was repeated.

Father had a real bad earache. This guy came to visit and told the old lady to make some cloth bags about six inches square and fill them with salt. He said Father was to put them in the oven to get them warm, then put one on a pillow and lie on it. When it got cold, he was to replace it with another one. After he did that for a while, a lot of liquid came out of the ear, and that was the end of the earache.

Other approaches. Sometimes flaxseeds were heated in the oven and placed in a cloth bag that was laid over the affected ear, or a raisin was heated and put inside the ear canal, or a piece of flannel was warmed and then tied around the ear and the forehead. The remedies listed above were repeated as often as was necessary.

Warm cow's milk and human breast milk were occasionally used to treat earaches. In the small town of Poultney, Vermont, I spoke with a farmer's wife.

I had lots of earaches when I was a child. A lady that lived down the road from us told me to come and sleep with her for the night. Every so often throughout the night, she squirted breast milk in my ear, and I haven't had another earache since that time.

NOSEBLEEDS

Cold. The most common way to deal with a bloody nose was to place a cold object on the back of the neck to constrict the blood vessels in the area. Because metals tend to retain the cold, items such as keys, scissors, and knives were often used. Cold water on a cloth was used in the same manner, and when ice was available it was wrapped in a towel and preferred over other remedies. Some felt that placing a cold object over the bridge of the nose was just as effective.

One lady recalled that there had been only one thing that would make her nose stop bleeding when she was a child: her mother would go into the cellar and pick out a rock that had been lying on the cold ground and hold it on the back of her neck.

A good-natured retired nurse lay in her hospital bed in the nursing home in Epsom, New Hampshire. (When our chat tired her out, she ended the interview by singing me a song.) This lady explained how she had treated nosebleeds.

> When a youngster's nose wouldn't stop bleeding, I would put several keys on a string and pull them up and down the child's back. You had to sneak up on the kid so he didn't know what was coming. He would tense up and go 'Ooooooh!' and it would make him shiver. In a few minutes the keys would be warm and the nose wouldn't be bleeding.

A similar tale was told:

> Two of my boys were playing baseball and they ran into each other. One of them got a bloody nose—my, how it did bleed! I didn't know how to stop it. It scared the daylights out of me, because I was alone except for the telephone, my savior.
>
> I called the doctor and he said to use shears on the back of the neck; if that didn't work, to use keys. The keys did the trick. In a short while, that clotted the blood.

A book of household hints published over a century ago states, "the sudden and unexpected application of cold is itself sufficient, in most cases, to arrest the most active hemorrhage. . . . For children, a key suddenly dropped down the back, between the skin and the clothes, will often immediately arrest a copious bleeding."[2]

Puffball spores. Some treated nosebleeds with puffball spores, a fine, silky-smooth powder that acted as a styptic.

A family would sometimes go out and gather all the puffballs they could find; they would break them open and store the powder in a jar. When the need arose, they would pack some into the nose for a speedy cure.

---

[2] Alexander V. Hamilton, *The Household Cyclopedia of Practical Receipts and Daily Wants* (Springfield: W. J. Holland and Co., 1874), p. 169.

Red material. Some people wore a piece of red yarn, string, or cloth around the neck to prevent nosebleeds; often a knot was tied in the front.

In Vermont, next to the Canadian border, I struck up a conversation with an elderly store clerk. When I explained my project, she was delighted to tell me about a remedy that had baffled her a few generations back.

> *My son had nosebleeds all the time. It was a real problem. You won't believe me, but my grandmother braided a red cord and put it on his neck, under his T-shirt so it wouldn't show, and it stopped the nosebleeds.*

Paper. Some had placed a piece of brown paper either on the roof of the mouth or between the teeth and upper lip to stop a nosebleed. This is one man's commentary on the treatment.

> *A nosebleed is caused by the house being too dry. You can squeeze your nose for fifteen minutes, but it's better to roll up a square piece of brown paper bag and place it between your teeth and upper lip. It stops it every time. White paper doesn't work—I've tried it.*

Another source told me that any kind of paper would do, even bathroom tissue.

Other approaches. Spiderwebs were sometimes packed into the nose. Some squeezed the nose for several minutes, while the head was held either down or back. Occasionally, raw salt pork was packed into the nose.

CANKERS, GUMBOILS, AND RECEDING GUMS

Goldthread root. I had never heard of goldthread until I started this project. Yet many seniors had used the roots of this plant, *Coptis trifolia,* for problems inside the mouth. Several said, "It was good for anything in the mouth." The plant's other names indicate its appearance and usefulness: yellow root, canker root, and mouth root. One didn't necessarily have to gather the roots, because many pharmacies sold them.

Goldthread root was popular for dealing with cankers and gumboils. Mostly, it was steeped and used as a mouthwash (repeatedly during the day), but a few chewed the root, or placed the root over the painful area.

> *Goldthread has a white star flower that blossoms in May. The leaf is like a shamrock, but bigger; the leaves are saw-toothed. The roots are a golden yellow—I would pick it in the spring, and I would pick it carefully, because the roots break if you just pull them up. I'd wash it, dry it, put it in a jar, and put it in the ice box. We used it on cankers. Boil it and slosh it around in the mouth.*

—

I'd go into the pine woods and gather yards and yards of goldthread roots. I'd dry it, and then make curls around my finger with it and store it in wax paper. I'd lay it over gumboils or cankers. It was very bitter to the taste so I wouldn't leave it in very long. After a while I'd put it in again.

It also makes the best cough syrup I ever had in my life: boil some up and mix it with sugar. I learned that from an old wood-chopper.

Many people I spoke with had used goldthread root on "sore mouth" and receding gums. Of these people, several had used it as a mouth rinse; a few had chewed the root.

For sore gums or cankers, I would pick goldthread root in the spring or summer in swampy woods. It's kind of like string and it looks like gold. It grows low to the ground in mossy, shady places. I would chew the root for a while, then spit it out. Keep repeating during the day until the gums are back to normal.

Some had used it in babies' mouths for teething and "sore mouth." It was swabbed on or used as a mouthwash.

Goldthread used to come in a small box. I would boil the roots in an earthen cup until the extract came out. Let it steep for about one hour and then cool it. For teething babies, I would dab the gums with a swab twice a day.

A few people mentioned using goldthread for a toothache, either bruising part of a root and packing it in a cavity, or chewing on it. One lady recalled that she'd had a tooth pulled and it wouldn't stop bleeding, so her mother had packed goldthread into the open gum.

Salt-water rinse. A solution was made by putting about a half-teaspoon of salt in one-half cup of warm water. The mouth was rinsed with the solution several times a day for various problems such as receding or bleeding gums, canker sores, tooth extraction, or toothache. Some still use this simple and cheap remedy.

A salt-water rinse is the best remedy. The salt firmed up the gums. It was the only preservative for meat—it keeps it firm. It does the same thing in your mouth. My dentist says it is the best antiseptic there is.

Alum. To treat a canker sore, many favored alum. Usually the powder was dabbed on several times a day, but some had taken a chunk of alum and rubbed it on. One lady who had used it on canker sores remarked, "Alum shrinks things."

TOOTHACHES

The standard toothache remedies our grandparents used could give only temporary relief. Before modern dental care was widely available, people suffered untold agonies from cavities.

My father was an alcoholic and my mother was a bootlegger; I have the still she used tucked away in the barn. There wasn't enough money to send us to a dentist. My teeth were rotten and I suffered with them for years.

———

We never told my stepfather that we had a toothache until the pain was unbearable. He had a blacksmith shop. He would set us under a kerosene lamp and take a pair of pliers that he had made and pull the tooth out.

———

If I had a loose first tooth that was giving me trouble, Mother tied one end of a string to the tooth and the other end to the doorknob of an open door. The string had to be taut. Then she would slam the door shut and the tooth made a rapid exit.

Cloves. People often used cloves and clove oil to treat a toothache. Some placed a few drops of clove oil on a piece of cotton and put it in the cavity or along the gums. Others applied the straight oil over the area. Crushed or powdered cloves were used in the same manner, and some simply put a whole clove on the affected tooth.

Put a cloth on the end of a toothpick and dab a drop of clove oil into the tooth. It stings real bad, but it sure makes the ache go away for a while.

———

For a toothache, we used oil of cloves. You've got to use a lot of it. Put it on cotton and place it along the tooth or in the cavity. It burned like the dickens. It would make the ache stop for two or three hours.

———

We'd take the head off a clove and put the end of the clove into the cavity. I don't know if it did any more than plug the hole and numb it a little bit.

———

Take a little bag made out of cheesecloth and fill it with ground cloves. Put it along the gums or in the tooth; or you can just sprinkle some of the powder over the tooth.

Interestingly, the shape of the clove is similar to that of a tooth, so herbalists would conclude that it would be useful for problems of the teeth. (The "law of signatures" holds that the shape, color, or a particular characteristic of a plant indicates the physical condition for which it is useful.)

Whiskey. Often, folks used whiskey to numb the pain of a toothache.

This really works. I'd use it to this day—if I didn't have false teeth. Buy the best whiskey you can get. Take some and hold it in the mouth on the tooth until it stops burning. Spit it out. The ache is gone for a few hours; then you do it over again.

———

I'd dip a piece of cotton batting in whiskey and bite on it until the pain was gone. It sort of anesthetized it. I used brandy on my son's gums when he was teething; he liked that the best. If he kept crying, I took a shot.

Salt. Several treatments used for a toothache involved the use of salt. Some gargled frequently with a warm salt-water rinse. Salt was heated on the stove or in the oven; it was placed in a cloth bag and applied to the face as a poultice. Salt, or a combination of salt and pepper, was put in the tooth cavity. Some rubbed salt on the gums.

Tobacco. Some chewed a wad of tobacco and placed it in the cavity. Others held a piece of tobacco leaf over the tooth. A few held tobacco smoke in the mouth for a period of time, and kept repeating the treatment.

Other approaches. Wintergreen oil was placed in the tooth, rubbed on the gums, or placed on cotton and held over the tooth. (Particular care was taken with children because small amounts could be toxic.) A used tea bag was placed on the tooth or along the gum. A cow-manure poultice was used externally.

A few of the uncommon remedies were particularly interesting.

Take the gray wall of a hornets' nest and soak it in vinegar. For a toothache, put that on the cheek as a poultice.

———

Pour vinegar on a plate and dunk brown paper in it. Take it out and sprinkle it with pepper. Put it right against your face and cover it over with a cloth. It felt so good; it was a lovely sensation, it made warmth and stopped the pain—I don't know how.

———

Cut an onion in half and put it on the pulse of the wrist on the opposite side that the ache is on, cut side down. Bind it on with a piece of sheet and leave it on overnight. The next morning, the ache is gone and the onion totally shriveled.

SORE THROAT

Dirty socks. At the inception of this project, a friend volunteered to introduce me to an elderly couple in Granville, Massachusetts. I readily accepted the offer and a few days later, we were en route. As we approached our destination, the muddy, potholed road hardly promised hospitality; but once the friendly couple welcomed us into their large, old farmhouse, the interview turned out to be well worth the trip. After a long discussion of other remedies, when we were getting ready to leave, I slipped in one more question: I wanted to know what they had done for a sore throat in years past.

The hefty gentleman started to chuckle and said that they used to tie a dirty sock around the neck.

In my ignorance, I assumed it was his idea of a bad joke, but when the expression on my face gave me away, he acted rather put out. No wonder! As I continued to interview people, it became clear that this was, in fact, a common practice across the Northeast.

There was a proper way to do it. A really dirty sock was used, preferably turned inside-out. The foot part of the sock was placed in the front, and so much the better if it was taken warm off the body.

Comments on this treatment were very similar.

For a sore throat, we'd wrap a dirty sock around the neck. I'd use my father's or brother's. All there were, were wool socks in those days. You'd wear them five or six days in a row—they didn't wash every day like they do now; had to wash by hand.

—

The most wonderful thing, you wouldn't believe it. We wore long, black stockings. We'd take a stocking that was still warm from wearing and wrap it around the throat. The smellier, the better.

—

I was a teacher, and some of my students used to come to school with the dirtiest stinking sock they could find wrapped around the neck. The smell was horrible.

—

When I had a sore throat, I would grease my throat with chicken fat or lard. Then I would take my mother's or father's warm, dirty sock and tie it around my neck before I went to bed. It really made me sweat.

Salt pork. To treat a sore throat, many people chose to place a long, thin strip of raw salt pork at the front of the neck and bind it on with a cloth. A common variation of this treatment was to sprinkle pepper on the salt pork and lay the peppered side against the neck.

The following stories give a better idea of how individuals used this treatment and its variations.

We got treated with salt pork. That cold against your neck was terrible. After a while, the grease would kind of lubricate. That salt pork, it done the trick.

—

For a sore throat, I'd take a strip of salt pork, less than half an inch thick. I'd lay it on a piece of flannel, put salt and sliced onions on it, and wrap it around my neck. I'd go to bed, and in the morning I wouldn't have no sore throat. The pork would be all withered and toughened and the onions would be black.

—

Take a thin slice of salt pork and sprinkle it heavily with pepper. Place against the front of the throat, and tie a dirty sock around it. Keep watching it so it doesn't burn.

—

When I had strep throat, Ma took salt pork and cut off two thin slices and covered them with pepper. Then she tied them on my throat. She didn't cover my windpipe. The next day, the strep was just about gone.

Kerosene. A popular sore-throat treatment was kerosene, and many people boasted of its effectiveness. Some placed a few drops on a teaspoon of sugar and ingested it; a few people told me they had taken a full spoon of the oil, unsweetened. Many chose to gargle with straight kerosene. One gentleman had learned the hard way that this was very dangerous: "I was gargling with kerosene and I accidentally swallowed some and it went down my windpipe. My lungs are scarred to this day."

I spoke with a nun who had been a missionary in Africa for sixteen years. Before she went there, she'd been given a course in basic, low-cost medical treatment. She described a variation on the kerosene remedy.

Put a tablespoon of kerosene in a small glass of lukewarm water and gargle with it. You can even swallow a sip. That remedy is nearly infallible.

Some other seniors spoke of different ways to administer the stuff.

One spoon of real kerosene oil, swallowed slow. Ma would say, "Don't hurry this." You'd swallow it slowly so it would lubricate your throat good. You could feel it open your throat right up.

—

I was given a teaspoon of straight kerosene at least once a day for sore throat. It didn't burn, but it tasted terrible and you couldn't wash it out.

One person recalled its external use, commenting, "Ma put kerosene on a rag and put it around my neck. That sore throat went right away, but I had a mess of blisters." Another source remembered kerosene being swabbed in his throat with a feather.

Oils. Various other oils were used to treat a sore throat. Somewhat popular was skunk oil, which was usually rubbed on the throat several times a day. Often it was covered with a piece of flannel or some other material. Some took it internally.

> *Eat one-half teaspoon of skunk oil for a tight sore throat. Some people put a little bit of salt on it to take away that greasy taste. It's even good for babies—give them a few drops. Too much would give you diarrhea.*

Butter was taken in a number of ways: one would eat a teaspoon of it warm, or drink a cup of hot milk with a chunk of butter in it, or even cream together butter and sugar and eat a spoonful.

Chicken fat and goose grease were rubbed on the throat, and some ate a small amount of either substance. One woman recalled having been treated with lard.

> *I remember when I was about ten years old and I had a sore throat. Mother put lard and pepper on a piece of brown paper bag and secured it to my neck. It was left on too long and it blistered my skin.*

> *I spent a lot of time over at Grandfather's house, and when I got better, I headed over there. He was a great poet; he could just look at you and make up a poem on the spot. (In World War I he was a seaman, and the boat he was on was torpedoed repeatedly by the German navy. He used to entertain the troops by making up rhymes.) When I got to his house I opened the door. He took one look at me and said,*

> > *"Gladys Pearl is a bonny girl*
> > *And she wears a bonny coat*
> > *She put black pepper on her neck*
> > *And blistered all her throat."*

Salt. Some chose to gargle periodically with warm salt water, the proportions generally being half a teaspoon of salt in a small glass of water. Some doctors still recommend this treatment:

> *Last year I went to the doctor with a sore throat. He said, "You have the medicine right at home, very cheap. A salt-water rinse, every half hour." In a couple of days, the throat was all right.*

One variation was a salt, baking soda, and warm water rinse.

> *One-fourth teaspoon salt, one-half teaspoon soda, and one-half glass of warm water. That was just as good as anything you could buy in the drugstore. Soda clears your throat out, and salt heals it up. They work together.*

Another remedy called for salt to be heated in a frying pan, placed in a small bag, and hung around the throat. One woman had her own version of the treatment: "We held a shovel of salt in the fireplace, filled a stocking with it, and tied it around the throat."

Sulfur. Sulfur was kept among the medicinals in many Yankee households. To treat a sore throat, some of our elders made a funnel out of a piece of paper and placed a pinch of sulfur in it. A second party would blow it into the throat. A spoon was sometimes used instead of paper, and one lady mentioned using a glass cylinder. A variation on this was to wet the tip of the finger, place sulfur on it, and stick the finger as far back into the throat as possible without causing the patient to gag.

In a church that serves as the senior center in Swanton, Vermont, I spoke with a lady who told me the following:

> When I was small, I had quinsy sore throat, and the doctor tried everything on me. Some old man used to come around the house for food and stuff; we called him Trampy. Most of us kids were afraid of him, but I guess he meant no harm. He would always bring us spruce gum to chew on.
>
> Grandma was talking to him and told him that my throat was all spotted with cankers. He told her to get some sulfur out. He took a wooden match and covered the bare end with a little piece of cotton batting (we didn't have swabs in those days). He wet it and stuck it in the sulfur. He put that sulfur right on the white spots, and those chunks of cankers came right off. Mom did the same thing a few times after that, and it healed up. I've used the same remedy on my own children more than once.

Vinegar. Some people had used a vinegar gargle several times a day. It was used straight, or in any of the following combinations:

> Vinegar and honey,
> Warm water and vinegar,
> Vinegar, warm water, and salt,
> Vinegar, warm water, and pepper.

One woman spoke of curing her own sore throat in a different manner:

> When my throat swelled, I poured a shotglass of vinegar, and added a little warm water and half a teaspoon of black or red pepper. I'd soak a cloth in it and put it into my mouth. The throat would go down.

Onions. For sore throats, some baked or boiled onions and wrapped them on the neck. One woman claimed that "A glass of milk with a finely chopped onion worked well." Some took onion syrup: often, an onion was sliced, placed in a bowl, and covered over with sugar. Below, a woman describes a different way of making onion syrup.

> Take a large onion and cut the top off. Scoop out the inside. Put sugar in it and place the top back on. Set it in the hearth on the coals until it's soft. When it's done, scoop out the juice in the center and cool it. Swallow some—it's great for sore throats.

Slippery elm. The inner part of the slippery-elm bark was sometimes used to soothe a sore throat. A grandmother from Hyannis, Massachusetts, explained, "It used to come in rough sticks and you would pull it apart. It tasted good, like anise."

Some had cooked the bark:

> Take the bark of the slippery elm and cook it slow. Then take off the slippery stuff with a knife. Add honey or sugar and take a spoonful as needed.

Sweet flag. Known to some as calamus, this plant has leaves similar to those of an iris, and it thrives in moist areas. Some Native Americans spoke favorably of the use of the roots of this plant for the treatment of sore throats. In Hogensburg, New York, one Mohawk tribe-member gave me a little chunk to chew on.

> We call sweet flag "holy root" in Indian. For a sore throat, chew a chunk of the root. It cools the throat and takes out the scratchiness. It also clears out sinuses and relieves any pressure in the head. You can also steep it and drink the tea. It has a pleasant, sort of bittersweet taste.
>
> It takes away evil spirits; I keep it on my windowsill. If you're drinking, chew it and they won't detect alcohol.

Other approaches. Honey was taken for a sore throat—either plain, mixed with lemon, or in hot tea. Some placed a few drops of turpentine on a teaspoon of sugar and ate it. Ginger tea and sometimes flaxseed tea were taken. A cold compress might be placed on the throat.

- 7 -

External Injuries

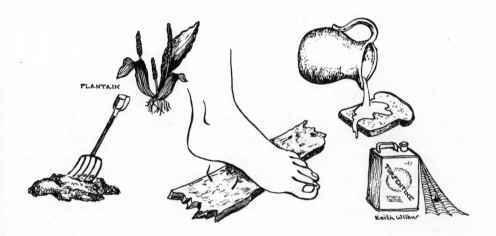

PLANTAIN

Keith Wilbur

BURNS

I had the good fortune of speaking to a Native American who sometimes gives lectures on Indian medicine. When I reached his home, I found him hosing down a large tub of fiddlehead ferns; he graciously took the time for a long chat. One of the things that interested me most was what he had to say about burns.

> When you get burned, you warm the area; when you put a burn under cold water, it's the worst thing you can do. If a person's feet were frostbitten, that person should not warm the feet up too quickly—because if they warmed too fast, the pain would drive him crazy and the skin might mortify. The same principle works in reverse for a burn; if it cooled too quickly, it would hinder the healing process.

Oils. I have a great deal of respect for Indian medicine, so I started to quiz seniors about the old-time practice of applying butter to burns. Since butter is noted for its ability to seal in heat, this would be consistent with what the medicine man told me. Did it work?

The reviews were mixed. Some people said flat-out that butter was no good, and a few even said it made a burn worse. But several people told me that butter would take away the burning sensation in a few minutes. One man said "It would take the burn out in half a day." Perhaps its effect depended on the severity of the burn.

Of the people who had used butter on burns, many felt it was effective *if* there was no salt in the butter, because salt would irritate the burn.

> *Put butter on burns and cover it over with flour. I made some frost-*
> *ing, cooked it on the stove. My daughter reached up and pulled it down on*
> *her face and chest. She was screaming—she has scars from it today. The*
> *butter takes a few minutes to stop the burning. Lard is better than butter*
> *because it has no salt in it—that's what my mother-in-law told me.*

> ———

> *When I was four years old, I lit a candle and put it in my side pocket,*
> *and the flame went up my arm. I was afraid to tell my mother right away*
> *because I knew she'd be mad. My mother plastered butter under my arm*
> *several times a day and bound it on with a cloth. My arm was up in the*
> *air for about five weeks. I got a good lickin' after I was cured.*

I was surprised to learn that, although butter was by far the most popular, many other different types of oils had been used.

> *When my son was three years old, I was preparing bath water. I had*
> *just poured boiling water into a tub on the floor and was about to pour in*
> *cold water when my son fell in head-first. His burns were very severe. All*
> *the skin came off, his face was all pus-like.*

> *I took about two cups of chicken manure and the same amount of pure*
> *lard. I boiled them together for about fifteen minutes, then let it cool. It*
> *makes a somewhat smelly yellow salve. I used it on him three or four*
> *times a day. In about two weeks he was healed, and no scar was left.*

> ———

> *For a light burn on the hand, hold your hand as close to the fire as*
> *you can. You can feel it drawing. It takes the pain out. You don't have to*
> *worry about tying it up, you can forget it. For a bad burn, we would put*
> *it in cold water, then put beef tallow on it and dust it with cornstarch.*

> ———

> *When I was five or six years old, Mother had a hot pail of mop water*
> *in the middle of the floor and she hadn't cooled it down yet. I backed into*
> *it. When my mother cut my clothes off, the skin came off my back. Moth-*
> *er, quick, got olive oil and poured it on my back. She had a roll of cotton*
> *and laid it over the oil and put me in bed. It hurt so. I had to lie on my*
> *stomach. Later on, when I went to bed for the night, she took the wet cot-*

ton off and put on fresh oil. She put cotton over that and then a thin nightie, a very soft, summer nightie.

I never had a scar, and it was healed in about a week. After the first few days, she did it once a day for a week. Never called the doctor, it just healed all up perfectly.

———

About seventy-five years ago, my father installed electricity. The maid had mopped the floor. You know, water and electricity don't mix. Mother plugged in the flatiron, and flame came up and covered her whole arm.

My father sent me to find the kerosene. It took me about ten minutes to find the can with the spout. My father poured kerosene all over the burn. Mother had to keep her hand flat in a pan so the kerosene would run into it. The doctor came over that evening to take a look at it, and there was no sign of a burn.

Other oils that were used on burns include bear's oil, chicken fat, goose grease, skunk oil, mutton tallow, cocoa butter, petroleum jelly, and fish oil.

This is another treatment that persisted over the centuries. The *Papyrus Ebers* contains a number of burn formulas that include oil.

Cold water. On the other hand, many people responded, "Never put butter on a burn, always immerse it in cold water." Some of these people were echoing modern-day physicians. Cold water keeps the pain at bay and greatly reduces the chance of infection. Flushing a burn with cold water is not a new practice; its roots are in the ancient past. In more recent literature, there are scattered references to this treatment, such as the following (from a medical book published in the last century): "Cold water is also excellent to apply, is always at hand, and can be used before any other means can be procured."[1]

When cold water is applied to a burn, it constricts the blood vessels and greatly reduces circulation on the area to which it is applied. This gives the cold-water treatment the advantage of anesthetizing a burn. By lowering the temperature of the "simmering" tissues, it minimizes the initial damage done.

Baking soda. There were folks who believed in applying baking soda to burns.

I was at a dinner party at a friend's house. The little girl burned herself on skewers that had meat on them. She started screaming. Baking soda was applied immediately, and within five minutes, the granddaughter was back at the table eating shishkabobs. It takes the heat out instantly.

———

[1] W. Beach, M.D., *The American Practice, Condensed; or the Family Physician* (New York: James McAlister, 1849), p. 603.

I've seen some terrible, terrible burns. It brings tears to your eyes to see the skin come off. The pulp mill caught fire in 1928. There was an explosion of "cooking liquor" and people were burnt with the acid. Chaos! The wall cracked up.

I worked in the pharmacy. For hours, we would take a spatula and mix bicarbonate with petroleum jelly in a big dish. We'd mix it up, and mix it up. . . . I'd bring it down in a big dish. We plastered patients with it.

We lost several people in the hospital. They brought a patient in on a stretcher, and he was dripping with acid. They had to make a new floor because it burned the wood right through. It was just like hell. There is nothing worse than a bad burn.

Other approaches. Burns were also treated with aloe vera, plantain leaves, cow-manure poultices, vinegar, a cold tea bag, a cloth soaked in cold tea, cold tea dabbed over the area, grated raw potato, slices of raw potato, or an egg-shell membrane.

I got a leg infection from a bad burn. The skin was white. I placed shredded raw potato over it as a poultice, and the next day the skin was a nice pink.

———

My baby fell out of the walker into the front of the heating stove. His eye and cheek were burned badly; the eye became sealed closed. I went to my neighbor and she told me to put eggwhite, one drop, right into the eye immediately, and to dab some over the entire burn. Soon after, he stopped crying.

Then I took the baby to the doctor; it was quite a ways. He said, "Hey, you don't need me, keep doing what you're doing—keep putting it on so it doesn't dry and crack."

SUNBURN

Vinegar. The remedy of choice for a sunburn was simply the application of vinegar. For those with delicate skin, the vinegar was watered down.

I have light skin and I used to sunburn very badly. I always got doused with vinegar after I came in from the sun. It worked well, but to this day, I won't eat anything with vinegar, even salads.

Other approaches. A few people mentioned applying grated raw potatoes or potato slices.

Put slices of raw potato over a sunburn. The starch in the potatoes comes out on your arm and leaves a whitish color. It feels so cool; gives a drawing sensation.

I spoke with a very delicate lady in Gloucester, Massachusetts, who had finally found a reliable source of relief by using an herbal tea.

Camomile is very good for a rash on the skin. Make a tea and wash it over your body. I went to a parade and was in the sun for three hours. I was very sick and couldn't sleep for two weeks. I was like a lobster. A lot of pain. I went to a special skin doctor. He said, "Lady, I never saw skin like yours. If you can get well, come in and tell me how you did it." I used cold camomile tea, sponged it on several times a day. In less than a week the burn went away.

CUTS, SLIVERS, AND EXTERNAL INFECTIONS

Salt pork. A popular way to treat a cut was with a poultice of some sort. One frequently mentioned practice was binding a thin slice of raw salt pork over the injured area; the application was changed daily. Many folks believed that if you used salt pork on a cut you would never get an infection. Some had used the application to pull out deep slivers, and a few reported that it would cure blood poisoning.

Salt pork was good on any bad cut. Cut a thin slice, place it on, and wrap it with gauze. It was a drawing agent; the salt pulls the pus out.

———

When my son was young, he was splitting wood and didn't take no caution—he cut the bottom of his foot. I put salt pork to the flesh with a bandage. He complained that the salt pork was making it burn. I used it on a leg wound once and it made it throb and beat.

———

When one of my boys was about fourteen years old, he was walking barefoot and stepped on some glass. The arch of the bottom of his foot was very painful. I poked around with a needle and couldn't find anything in the foot. I took him to the doctor's and he couldn't find anything; said it wasn't there. I said, "There's got to be."

My son would cry something terrible because it hurt so. I applied a salt-pork poultice, a fresh one every day. Even with the poultice, it would hurt him so. After about a month, about an eighth of an inch of glass came out of the surface. I took him back to the doctor and had him pull the glass out: it was like a pyramid, almost an inch long.

One lady recalled simply using the brine:

We always had a barrel of salt-pork brine in the cellar. If we cut our hand, we'd take a cup of it and pour it over the cut. We would dance around for a while after it, because it stung something wicked. But it healed fast.

Bread and milk or water. Poultices of bread and milk had many advocates; a few had used bread and water. This poultice was used to stop bleeding, heal infections, and draw slivers, and it was occasionally used to treat blood poisoning. One old gent told me he had refused to eat bread pudding when he was growing up because he thought he would be eating a poultice.

A bread-and-milk poultice was a standard remedy in our household for a splinter in the finger, or an infection in a cut. We always kept it on until it was dry. Canned milk worked better than regular. They were hard to bandage up—it was a glob. It would get hard and smell sour.

———

A bread-and-milk poultice brings things to a head. It will make a splinter come up. Break up the bread and put milk in it and heat it on the stove. Squeeze the milk out and put it on as warm as you can stand it. It's the heat that draws.

———

I was cutting wild edibles for the chickens, and I had to cut them up fine. I didn't want to do it in the worst way. I cut my thumb real bad—here's the scar. Mother grabbed a piece of bread, dunked it in water, and slapped it on my thumb. She changed the poultice three or four times a day. It stopped the bleeding and saved the tip of my thumb.

Manure and urine. Several people reported that fresh manure (usually cow manure) made an effective poultice for cuts, slivers, infections, and blood poisoning. In Berlin, New Hampshire, an old farm gal told her story.

My husband was out in the pasture doing butchering with his boss when he got a deep cut. He had no chance to clean it, infection set in, and he got blood poisoning.

We took some fresh cow manure and heated it up in the kerosene stove in the shed, because we didn't want to stink up the whole house. You put it on as hot as you could stand it. Put it in a towel and wrap it around the hand. The next morning, all the blood poisoning was out and the swelling was down.

———

We lived on a farm. My sister, when she was a young girl, she carved her boyfriend's initials in her arm, then she filled it in with ink. It got infected and turned into blood poisoning. Red lines went up the arm. The doctor didn't know what to do; he was going to cut the arm off. Fresh, warm cow manure was put on it, and the next day it was better.

———

For a bad infection, we would make an animal-dung poultice—deer, cow, horse, any grass-eaters. Take manure, add some water, boil it five to ten minutes, and cook until mushy. Put it on warm and cover it. There's lots of heat in horse manure, twice as much as any other kind. Change the poultice once a day. It draws the poison out.

—

Fresh cow manure or horse manure stops bleeding. I was chopping wood; the axe fell on the instep. I bound manure on it and it stopped bleeding within five minutes.

Some people I interviewed had used urine on cuts to prevent infections. In a nursing home in Roscoe, New York, a nurse's aide told me the following:

Brother and Dad were out logging deep in the woods. He was seventeen at the time. A log came down on his head. He got a good gash—which didn't seem to bother him. But he came home just furious because Dad peed on his head. He was just furious that Dad did that. All he could talk about was the urine.

Pitch and turpentine. A wad of pine pitch was sometimes placed over a cut to stop bleeding. It was also used to remove slivers and to treat and prevent infections. One person referred to this as a "woodsman's remedy" because it was such convenient first aid for lumberjacks, trappers, and others who worked in the forest.

They'd put pine pitch on cuts. It would dry out and was just like tar. It was hard to wear off; you couldn't wash it off.

—

If you're out in the woods with an axe and you cut yourself, put a glob of pine pitch on the cut and that stops the bleeding. It will draw poison out, and heal a cut right up.

In Baxter Park, Maine, a camper told me the following story:

My neighbor found a shot doe. He plugged the wound with pine pitch and bound it on with a rag. He put a collar around the deer. The deer was two or three years old when he found her. She healed and followed him around. He had the deer for two years, then she went back to the wild. Some time later, he spotted her with other deer; they all ran but her. She stood and gazed at him for a moment, then she ran too.

A few people mentioned having applied turpentine to cuts.

Turpentine was my dad's favorite remedy for cuts. I fell over a rusty barbed-wire fence one day and got two good gashes. He poured turpentine over it—did it burn and smart! I wouldn't speak to him for about a week. I thought the cure was worse than the cut.

Plantain. Some of our elders reported that the common plantain, *Plantago major*, was highly effective when used on cuts, external infections, splinters, and blood poisoning. Use of this plant in early American and British medicine also indicates that it was considered a potent medicine. *The Medical Herbalist,* published in the 1930s, states, "The plant is considered specific against the bites of a mad dog or venomous creatures." [2]

A tiny, wiry, ninety-year-old lady from Northampton, Massachusetts, told the following story:

> When I was a child I was out in the woods picking blueberries and I was bit by a garden snake. I'd heard that if a snake bites you, you should cut the bite and squeeze the blood out, so that's what I did. The knife wasn't sterile and I got blood poisoning. My foot doubled in size. The doctor wanted to cut my leg off, but my mother said, "Hell, no!"
>
> As soon as the doctor left the house, she started to treat me with plantain leaves. She would heat the leaves on the stove with an iron, put them on the leg and foot hot, and tape them on. When the leaves cooled, she'd put on a new batch. It drew the poison out and the leg was fine in a few weeks.

Other people told how they had used plantain:

> Plantain is antiseptic. A little kid fell and gashed his forehead. The medicine woman chewed plantain, placed it on the wound, and tied it on with a hankie. It's also good for a bee bite.

> ⎯

> Plantain is good for any infection, anything with pus—cuts, boils, eye infection. First apply butter, not margarine, then the leaves. Wrap and leave on for twenty-four hours.

> ⎯

> For cuts, open sores, or infections, take plantain leaves and drop them into boiling water for a few minutes until they're wilted. Place the hot leaves on the cut, wrap, and leave on. Do this three times a day—it will draw out pus, wood, or briar.

One man recalled the time he'd had an infected cut on a finger and wrapped plantain around the entire digit. He said it had gotten worse, because "it was drawing on both sides of the finger."

There are several varieties of plantain in New England, all considered equally effective. The ovate green leaves grow from a central whorl; each leaf has several noticeable veins that go from stem to tip of the leaf. If you live in the Northeast, the probability is high that plantain grows in your yard.

Spiderwebs. Some folks found spiderwebs to be an effective styptic and healing agent for cuts.

[2] J. R. Yemm, editor, *The Medical Herbalist,* vol. XI, The National Association of Medical Herbalists of Great Britain, Ltd., 1937, p. 61.

For a cut or wound, you would stick your finger in a web and make circles. Then you'd make a ball and pack it into the cut, and it stopped the bleeding. The yellow dots on the web were the best.

———

Take a fresh loaf of rye bread and pull out a dab from the loaf. Knead it with spiderwebs and apply it to the cut. To gather webs, put a pillow case over the top of a broom and sweep the corners of the ceiling.

———

Webs will stop bleeding quicker than anything. Don't bandage them on. We used them especially on animals; when we cut off a cow's horns, we put cobwebs on to clot the blood.

———

Grandpa's pipe set the house on fire. I put my hand through a windowpane trying to get out. I broke the glass and got a deep gash. Father got webs off the beams in the barn and stuck them in the cut. It coagulates the blood in a severe cut.

———

I cut my thumb and I couldn't stop it from bleeding. An old woman got a glob of spiderwebs from the cellar beams and packed it in. That stopped the bleeding. You'd think you'd get infected from that dirty stuff, but you never did.

Puffballs. Yankees also used the spores from puffballs to stop bleeding. This is one of many areas in which allopathic medicine and folk medicine converged. In the past, doctors used this substance during surgery for the same purpose.

I had the mumps and I got out of bed to get something to drink in the kitchen. I started to pass out and took hold of the tablecloth. I pulled it down and a dish came off and cut my nose. I couldn't stop it from bleeding, so I put some puffball powder on it, then I went back to the bedroom and lay down. Mother said, "What happened in the kitchen, did the cats do that?"

———

I was in an accident and a bone in my wrist came out through the skin—got about a three-inch scar. I put puffball spores on it and it stopped the bleeding until I could get to a doctor.

Alum. Some treated cuts with alum. (Alum styptics are used to stop the bleeding from razor cuts.) An active eighty-year-old woman in Bellows Falls, Vermont, spoke almost in a whisper as she told the following:

My mother would clean the top of the stove real good and put a chunk of alum on top. It would bubble up and blister and spread out like a pancake. Then she would take the griddle off the stove and let it cool, then powder it up.

Dad was always chopping wood, and a few times he cut himself. Once he got a deep cut on the leg. My mother took a piece of paper and made a tube and blew some alum into the cut.

We also used it when a horse's leg was half cut off. The vet said it would never heal. He was our pet. We washed the leg with peroxide and put alum on it every day. It healed. It also kept the flies away.

Other approaches. There were many other applications used on cuts and external infections. Some of them were the membrane from inside an eggshell, aloe, witch hazel, sugar, a raw-potato poultice, and a flaxseed poultice. Some people soaked the injured area in Epsom salts and warm water; a few reported this would cure blood poisoning. Occasionally, tobacco leaves were used.

My dad used to make snowshoes. His knife was so sharp we were never supposed to touch it. I had my sister hold up a piece of cowhide leather so I could cut it. I got cut and was bleeding like mad. Father got a tobacco leaf from the neighbor and put it over it to stop the bleeding. It was bleeding so much—but I was more scared of my father than the blood.

PUNCTURE WOUNDS

Salt pork. In rural areas, it was not uncommon to step on a rusty nail or even to have a pitchfork land on the foot. To avoid getting the dreaded lockjaw (tetanus) and to avoid infection and blood poisoning, a high percentage of people treated their puncture wounds with salt pork. This was a surprisingly simple remedy, given that tetanus killed many of its victims, and in a most insidious manner.

A thin slice of raw, all-fat salt pork was bound over the puncture with a cloth (a few had used the rind). Most people changed the application daily and continued the treatment until the soreness went away.

When you step on a rusty nail, slap on a piece of salt pork and keep walking. Change it every day until the soreness goes away, usually three or four days. Salt draws the poison right out.

———

My husband stepped on a nail, and his foot became infected. I took the salt pork off at the end of each day to change it and make sure the red rings around the wound were getting lighter. The poison would come out on the rind and color it. The skin would turn a delicate pink where it had been red.

———

I was raspberrying. I stepped on a nail and it almost went clear through the foot. It happened to be the day the meat man would come, Wednesday. His name was Lesmore. Mother got salt pork from him. When she took it off my foot, it was all green. It took all the poison out of my foot.

———

I slipped off a sloped roof and fell on a spike, punctured my leg. Got blood poisoning. I put a slice of salt pork over it and headed for the doctor's. Old Doc Branch had a very deep voice; he said, "That works very well, pulls the dead blood and everything out."

———

There were eight kids in our family. In the summer we were encouraged not to wear shoes because it would wear them out. Pitching hay, sometimes one of us would get a puncture. We would put a salt-pork poultice over it and leave the same one on for three days. The grease seemed to make the wound soft and keep it open.

———

When my daughter was five years old, a collie bit her on the face: there was a puncture mark on the left cheek and one on the jaw. I remembered that Mother had said that salt pork was good for everything, so I put some over the bite. That evening the doctor came over and told me, "That's a good old-time remedy." To this day, people think it's a dimple, they don't realize it's a scar.

Our grandparents certainly had a great deal of faith in the medicinal value of salt pork. They believed it would pull out any type of poison. Although this treatment was reported to be very effective, we should keep in mind that the salt pork used was usually taken right out of the brine; it was probably more potent than the salt pork we buy today.

One source remembered that his friend got into trouble when he wrapped salt pork around the entire foot. He said it "worked against itself." (In the section on cuts, a similar comment was made about plantain.) The drawing power on both sides may have locked in the poison and neutralized any positive effect.

Manure poultice. A distant second in popularity in my collection was the manure poultice—usually cow manure.

Father was doing chores in the barn; a rusty nail ran into his heel. Before long, several streaks went up his leg: streaked to his groin. It was out in the country and Mother didn't dare leave him. She took a big, old eight-quart milk pan, ran to the barn, and got fresh manure right from the drop, and put Father's foot in there. Then she went to fetch the doctor; he came over after office hours.

The manure began to work right away, it pulled the poison down. The manure made it burn like the dickens, it kept burning; it was like a drawing sensation. The next morning, it was all gone, and the doctor told Mother she saved Father's life.

———

There was a fella from down on Cobb Street who came into my father's store, and he had one boot on. I said, "One boot?" He said he had a poultice in there made from horse manure to draw the poison out because he'd stepped on a nail. This was about seventy-five years ago. . . . He thought that manure was really great. He felt the heat would draw out the poison.

Bread-and-milk poultice. Some Yankees used a bread-and-milk poultice, alone or in combination with other substances.

A nail went into my foot. Ma used a warm bread-and-milk-and-nutmeg poultice. You mush it up good and pack it on both sides of the hole. I swear it was the yeast that made it work.

———

When I was about six years old, I was visiting my cousin on the farm. They were cleaning up the old hog pen and there were boards all over the ground with spikes in them. I was barefoot. A large spike went completely through my foot. Mother put a cold bread-and-milk poultice directly over the sore, and catnip leaves over that. It was changed a few times a day, and left on all the time until the swelling went down.

Hair smoke. The following story was told by a lady whose grandmother had gotten tetanus and been fortunate enough to recover.

My grandmother would often tell the tale of how she got a very deep rusty nail puncture that wouldn't heal. She was very sick for two months. It was summer and her mother would bundle her up and put her in the sun, and still she had chills. Nothing worked.

A band of gypsies came around because her mother used to feed them. A gypsy woman said, "I will heal it if you will let me." The gypsy woman took a felt hat and put it on fire and put it under the wound to let the smoke go into it for about ten minutes. It stopped the pain almost immediately. She did it three or four times a day and my grandmother was healed in a few days.

A lady from Skowhegan, Maine, told of a similar method that was used in her family for prevention of lockjaw.

> *Father had fifty cows, ten horses. The hired help were always stepping on nails. Mother would place a wool rag on the hot coals in the kitchen range and hold the foot right over the burning rag so the smoke would go in it. She claimed it was the fumes from the wool, the lanolin, that worked. Then she'd put on a slice of salt pork.*

The following comment suggests that lanolin may have special properties.

> *The still-current wisdom among sheep farmers is that the lanolin that coats a sheep's wool and skin is a natural antiseptic and blood-stop when an unfortunate sheep happens to get nicked by the shearer. It is true; they do stop bleeding almost right away, and the cuts heal within just three days or so.*

Other approaches. Puncture wounds were also treated with turpentine, a wad of chewed tobacco, plantain leaves, or a brown-soap-and-sugar poultice.

BEE AND WASP STINGS

When a bee or wasp stings, it injects a small amount of formic acid, which usually causes irritation or localized swelling. Some people, though, are allergic to this substance, and some have died within half an hour of a sting. Anyone who is allergic needs quick medical attention.

In treating a sting victim, the first consideration is to remove the stinger; if it is left in, it will keep pumping venom for a few minutes.

Mud. Yankees had numerous ways to proceed after removing the stinger, but the most common by far was the application of mud. If the soil was too dry to hold together, saliva or water was mixed in with the earth to get it moist enough to apply.

An elderly lady from the college town of Amherst, Massachusetts, remembered the time when she was six years old and at a picnic with her family at Mountain Park.

> *I climbed up a birch tree unsuspectingly, and there was a hive of bees. They came under my dress and every inch of me was stung. I ran from the bees, and my grandmother said for everyone to spit into the hard earth to make mud. As soon as the mud was applied to the bites, I got relief. If you get it on right away there is no swelling.*

A severely arthritic little lady recalled an incident from her childhood:

> *I got stung on my finger, and my father told me to dig a small hole in the ground and stir my finger in it for a while. After that, the swelling went away.*

It is noteworthy that some of our forefathers felt that swamp mud offered the most effective cure for insect stings:

> *For a bee bite, put on rich, black mud from a swamp where there are layers of mud and decaying leaves. It will absorb the venom.*

Baking soda. A thick paste of baking soda and water was often used to neutralize insect stings. Some people still rely on this remedy. There were some who left out the water and made the paste with rubbing alcohol, vinegar, or ammonia.

One grandfather believed that the following remedy was effective when used by people with allergies, who were not able to get to the doctor quickly: "In a half a cup of water, dissolve a teaspoon of baking soda, a half a teaspoon of vinegar, and a little sugar; mix and drink."

Other approaches. The following substances were also applied to a sting: a slice of raw onion, a wad of chewed tobacco, a flaxseed poultice, a paste of salt and water, vinegar, ammonia, rubbing alcohol, turpentine, and witch hazel.

- 8 -

Skin Conditions

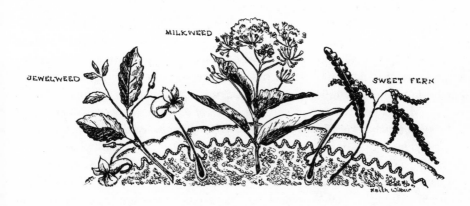

JEWELWEED · MILKWEED · SWEET FERN

BOILS AND CARBUNCLES

A boil begins with a bacterial infection at the root of a hair. As pus collects, the surrounding area becomes swollen and painful. We seldom hear of a case of boils anymore; yet they were once common.

A retired Yankee threadgrinder with whom I spoke keeps busy in the summer months growing and selling some of the nicest gladioluses and bouquets of cut flowers in his area. Although he is seventy-two years old, each year his garden expands. He recalled the time when boils were a frequent scourge.

> *When I was in high school, it was like an epidemic; we got them most-ly on the neck, but they sometimes popped up on the butt and in the odd-est places. It seems like before and after that period, people seldom had boils. I don't know what caused it.*

The carbuncle is a compound, multi-cored boil. Sometimes a large carbuncle would keep a person bedridden for weeks. *The Library of Health*, written in 1920, states, "the pain and exhausting discharge wears out the strength so much that it may cause death; if a second of large size appears, after the first begins to heal, as it is not very unusual, it quite frequently proves fatal." [1]

Flaxseeds. A poultice made of flaxseeds was a favorite treatment for bringing a boil or a carbuncle to a head and drawing out the foul matter. When making a flaxseed poultice, old-timers would grind about a tablespoon of the seeds and then boil them in a little water until the liquid turned gelatinous. The eruption would then be covered with a clean cloth, the mush spread over it as hot as could be tolerated, and the whole dressing covered with another cloth. Some chose to make a neater poultice by placing the mixture in a small cheesecloth or flannel bag. In either case, it would be left on for an hour or two, usually until it dried, and the process would be repeated at intervals during the day until the eruption came to a head and the pus was drawn out.

> *My brother had a large boil on the back of the neck. It was so bad he couldn't turn his head from side to side. My mother boiled flaxseeds until it became a thick pudding. She put the seed-mixture in a small cheese-cloth bag and applied it to the boil. In one hour it came to a head; a few hours later, he could move his neck again.*

Linseed oil. Linseed oil is pressed from flaxseeds; it was sometimes heated and used in the same manner as the flaxseed poultice.

> *I used to get a siege of boils. Mother would heat up some linseed oil and apply it to the boils as a poultice. She'd put a cotton cloth on the boils, linseed oil, and then another piece of cloth. She'd leave it on for a while, until the heat was out of it, and then apply a new one, as hot as I could stand it.*

Cupping. One lady explained another method that people had used to deal with boils. (This is one remedy that one was not likely to forget.)

> *If I remember correctly, it would take a boil a week to ten days to come to a head. When it was ripe, you would place a small bottle in a pan and boil it for a few minutes. You would pick it up with tongs or a pot-holder and dump the water out of it. Then you'd place the neck of the bottle over the boil. It worked so fast, the suction would pop the boil and the stuff would ooze out. It would leave a little red ring from the bottle neck.*

> *I had a boil on my arm; it came to a point. You know, that sucker wouldn't break. I put hot water in a bottle, dumped it out and put the top of the bottle over the boil. So much pain, I almost died—but it pulled the core and all the pus right out.*

[1] Frank B. Scholl, Ph.G., M.D., *Library of Health* (Philadelphia: Historical Publishing Co., 1920), p. 716.

When that thing popped, it was almost like blowing your head off.
The first time, you didn't know what was coming. But after that, you
didn't want it done again.

One lady's face evidenced her aversion as she recalled the process, noting she had "passed out like a light" when it was done to her. Another commented, "It sucked the boil out, but it pretty near killed me. It was brutal, especially if you had a boil on your bottom."

Yellow lye soap. Another treatment for a boil or carbuncle was to take a bar of yellow lye soap and to scrape off a small amount. The scrapings would then be mixed with a dab of water and a little bit of sugar, either brown or white, or molasses. The concoction would be bound on and changed a few times a day until the eruption came to a head. Consensus held that this mixture had strong drawing qualities.

I had big boils all down my left arm and on my chest. In the very mid-
dle of a boil is a green thing like a stem, about a quarter-inch long. Once
that core is out, it heals up. I would soften a piece of yellow soap, mix in a
little sugar, put it on the boil, and bandage it on. After four or five hours,
the core is right in the soap.

One lady spoke of an uncommon variation of this treatment:

I had boils on the back of my neck. Take a little water and put in a
piece of white soap. Bring it to a boil; it will make suds. Put cornmeal in
it to make a soft poultice. It draws the head right out so slick and clean
you'd never know you had the boil. It healed right up afterwards.

Bread-and-milk or water. Bread-and-milk poultices, and occasionally bread-and-water poultices, were used to treat boils and carbuncles. (An occasional old textbook will mention bread-and-water poultices.)

I had a boil on my neck and it was paining me dreadful. Mother
soaked bread in milk and tied it around my neck; it was left on overnight.
The boil came to a head in the morning, and I had bread and milk all over
my hair.

———

Fifty-three years ago, I had a carbuncle above my waist on my right
side. [She showed me a good-sized scar.] My mother knew a lot of reme-
dies, but I didn't dare tell her or the doctor because I was afraid of what
either of them might do. It had become quite painful, and one night my
husband put his foot down and said it was time to treat it.

As soon as I crawled into bed, he mixed red hot water with bread and
put it in a linen bag and placed it on, real hot. The pain was so bad, I
thought I would pass out. To this day, when he looks back on it, he says
that he was cruel to me that night.

By morning, the poultice had brought it way out. It was red and ugly, about three inches in diameter and about two inches deep. You could have put a golf ball in there and lost it. At that point, my husband insisted that I go to my mother or a doctor. After I saw the doctor, the nurse came over every day and pushed around the sides to get the pus out. Then she would paint it with a colored solution. A few times, she got a mugful of pus out of it. I had a month of hell. I'd rather have a baby any day than go through that again.

Other approaches. A salt-pork poultice or an egg-shell membrane was sometimes applied to boils. Three methods were used to purify the blood to get rid of boils: some ate a small box of raisins daily; some ate a yeast cube a day; and others took sulfur and molasses for several days in a row. Nutmegs were occasionally used.

I used to have a lot of boils. I was really full of them. I had them under my arms, in the buttocks, and in my private parts. I used to have to walk with my legs apart. It was more like a shuffle. I even jumped rope with my legs apart. I was just a little kid, but I suffered so that I can remember it.

Mother and Grandmother sat down at the kitchen table and discussed what to do about it. They decided to put a hole in a nutmeg and put a shoestring through it and make a necklace. I wore it down low so no one could see it. In about six weeks the boils were gone. I don't know if the nutmeg cured them or not.

———

I had an awful lot of boils and carbuncles on the back of my neck. A young schoolteacher said, "Take a nutmeg, and any time you think of it, bite off a little piece and chew it." So I carried one in my pocket. Every half hour or hour, I took a bite. You need good teeth, though. It seemed to do the trick.

I spoke with a square-jawed, sharp-witted lady who was in her hundredth year. She sat in her rocking chair in a country nursing home and related the following story:

My father had a carbuncle on the back of his neck that wouldn't break. The doctor had tried everything. He was almost crazed with the pain and they were about to take him to a sanatorium. An old Indian woman who was a friend of the family offered to help. She took a dish towel and went to the barn and filled it with fresh cow manure and then she placed it on the carbuncle as a poultice. My father dozed off for about half an hour. When he woke, most of the pain was gone, and he mowed lawn that afternoon.

A man from Willimantic, Connecticut, recalled a harsh treatment that he had used.
I had plenty of boils. I took wood ashes and mixed them with water and made a plaster. You don't bind it on. I changed it a couple of times a day. It was tough medicine but it drew them out.

OPEN SORES

Resins. People spoke of numerous substances used to treat open sores, but only one class of substance could be called popular: the resins from various pine trees. Some were partial to pitch from the white pine, others had used balsam fir, and a few said it didn't matter what type of conifer the resin came from.

In this department, the grandfathers have a monopoly on the stories.

Take any pine tree and make a V in the tree so the pitch will run down. Catch it in the summertime when it's really warm—it's the only time it will run. Put it in a can. For a sore or a splinter, put pitch on it and cover it over. Leave it on overnight. The pitch draws it out.

———

Take pine gum and put it in a container. It will harden up. You use it on an infected sore that won't get clean. You heat it up a little with the tip of a knife, put it on the sore, and cover it over.

———

Collect pine pitch from a white pine log. Heat the pitch until it's watery, then strain it through a cloth. Mix that with petroleum jelly or animal fat (but the animal fat tends to spoil)—use half petroleum jelly, half pine pitch. You can keep it in a jar. It's good for sores, cuts, festers, any infection.

———

We used pine pitch for all kinds of healing: it has a wonderful drawing effect. Every fall, Father would collect a whole jar of it.

Mother had a sore on her side, and put some pitch on it and covered it over with a cloth. She left it on overnight. It turned out to be an internal abscess. The pitch drew it to the hole, but the hole was not large enough for it to come out. It was very painful because the pus was forming underneath. The doctor had to lance it.

———

We applied balsam-fir pitch to sores. Find a blister on the tree, place a bottle under it, and prick it: the pitch would flow into the bottle. The squaws would make a salve out of it that was good for anything.

A few people mentioned using a different kind of resin on open sores, that from the buds of balsam poplar. They were soaked for a few days in rubbing alcohol or liquor. The buds were then strained out and the resulting solution was called balm of Gilead. The solution was applied to open sores several times a day.

Other approaches. Also used were salt-pork poultices, plantain leaves, yellow soap mixed with sugar, flaxseed poultices, bread-and-milk poultices, and dry or wet cornstarch. Other treatments were also mentioned.

The doctor wanted to cut my husband's legs off—he had a kind of cancer, a hole like a half-dollar in the middle of the front of each leg. You could see into the holes. It was caused by sugar diabetes. I wouldn't allow the doctor to cut the legs off.

As soon as I brought him home, I started to work on it. I would dissolve cornstarch and pour it in. I did it three times a day. It took three weeks to save his legs. It didn't start to heal until his bowels let go.

—

My brother came to visit. I said to him, "What's that terrible smell?" It was a leg ulcer, and he had been going to the doctor for over a year with it. I told him to go out into the shed and bring a clean handkerchief with him, to gather a bunch of spider webs and place them on the ulcer and wrap it with the hankie. I told him to change it every day. The ulcer healed within a month.

—

A friend of mine had a leg ulcer and she used to send her sister out at night to get fresh mullein leaves from the pasture. They had to be fresh so the sticky stuff was still on them. They would wrap the leg in them, changing them often and through the night. They were secured on but not bandaged, because air was good for the sore. When you removed the leaves, they would be all black.

—

Aloe would heal sores. My aunt fell down a flight of stairs and skinned the front of her leg and couldn't get it healed. (There was diabetes in her family; she might have had it too.) This went on for quite a while. Aloe took care of it.

—

For sores, there's nothing better than bleach. I had blood and pus in my heel; I tried everything on it. Finally, I used hot water with a little bleach. Soaked my foot in it three times a day for about twenty minutes and that did it.

———

Camomile is wonderful for animals. My cat got into a fight and got a horrible leg infection. The vet couldn't clear it up and told me it was always going to run. I made a very strong camomile tea and took a cotton ball and squeezed some of it into the wound. I would hold it on for a few minutes, and do it at least three to four times a day. In two weeks, the cat was walking on all fours again.

COLD SORES

Alum. The favorite remedy used to treat cold sores was alum, either powdered or a small chunk that could be rubbed on the lesion. It was used a few times a day.

I would use a little chunk of alum. It would look like a rock. I'd rub some on. It would pucker your lips for a few minutes. It draws real hard. The cold sore would go away in a day or so. Grandpa used it when he shaved to stop the bleeding.

———

We dabbed on powdered alum two or three times a day. It dried up the cold sore, took the scab right off. It tastes terrible—it curls the tongue to the top of the head.

Camphorated oil and camphor ice. Some treated cold sores by rubbing them frequently with camphorated oil or camphor ice. These preparations reportedly had drawing powers. One lady remarked, though, "Camphorated oil works for some, for others it will spread the cold sores."

Other approaches. A few people mentioned applying aloe vera gel several times a day to heal cold sores. A handful of people had rubbed earwax over cold sores.

A woman came to me with cold sores all over her face. I told her to put her finger in her ear and rub the wax all over them. Once a day. In five days, her face was clear. It's also good for badly cracked lips.

WARTS

Rituals. The most popular way to remove warts was to take an object such as a dishrag, a bean, a potato peel, or a piece of salt pork or bacon, rub it on the wart, and bury it in the ground. It was believed that when the object had rotted, the wart would be gone. Some people expressed the opinion that the object must be stolen or the process would not work. Some would rub an object on the wart and then throw it over the left shoulder; it was important not to look to see where the object had fallen.

It might seem that our elders were half-crazed, using some of these amusing remedies; but the fact is, many warts can be cured by hypnotism and self-hypnotism. Confidence in such rituals could indeed work. Another consideration is that warts result from viral infection and often disappear spontaneously over a period of time.

The following is a sampling of other rituals used to remove warts.

When I was a little kid, I had warts on my hands. I went outdoors early in the morning and rubbed my hands through the dew on the ground. I only did it that one time, but it worked.

—

Got rid of a big seed wart on my hand. The old man at the little general store said, "I can get rid of that for you." He scraped a little salt pork and put it on. In three weeks it was gone. The poor guy went to Florida, came back, and died of a heart attack before I got a chance to tell him.

—

Grandma had a boarding house and these people came to get a room. They said to Mother, "What's the matter with the kid? She's got so many warts on her hands." Mother said that I'd always had them. The woman said to her husband, "Why don't you take them off?"

He cursed them while he spit on his finger, then rubbed two fingers together. Then he rubbed the index finger on a wart, wiped the two fingers on his pants, and started all over again. He jibber-jabbered all the while so I couldn't understand him. All the warts went away except the one that I had used to show my friends how he had done it.

—

There is magic in warts. My brother-in-law could take warts off. I don't know how he done it. He counted the warts on me—I had seventeen. He made a knot in a piece of yarn for each wart and then buried the yarn in the ground. He told me that in two weeks they would be gone, and they were.

—

This stands out very vividly in my mind. When I was a little girl, not more than four years old, I had warts all over my hands. They were unsightly and Mother didn't like the looks of them. When Grandma died, the casket was left in the house. It was placed near the marble fireplace and it had a big fur rug in front of it.

I didn't know Grandma was dead; I thought she was asleep. My aunt and Mother were standing next to the casket and I heard my aunt say, "I'm sure Ma would have wanted you to do it." I can remember them holding me up and putting my two hands on Grandma's forehead and saying, "Grandma is cold." When they put me down, they told me that the warts would soon disappear. Sometime later, they were gone.

Even some doctors were involved in this hocus-pocus.

My daughter had seed warts, so I took her to the doctor. He gave her a salve to rub on them and then asked me to leave the room. He whispered to her, "You go home and get some dried beans. Rub a bean over each wart and then hide them down deep in a bag of flour and don't tell anyone. When your mother finds the beans, the warts will be gone."

One day I was sifting flour and I found the beans in it. I asked my husband and the boys about them, then I asked Mary. First she looked down at her hands and saw the warts were gone, and then she confessed she'd done it and explained why.

A Vermont lady had several warts, one of which was very annoying. She told me she had solved the problem when she "sold the warts to Mrs. Blackadar for a nickel and they went away." The following is a sampling of other rituals that were used: some carved a cross on a willow tree for each wart; food was rubbed on the warts and thrown outdoors, since it was believed that the animal that ate the food would get the warts; a blade was rubbed through the twig of an apple tree, and then the blade was rubbed on the warts.

Rituals were occasionally used for other conditions. One man recalled the time he had a wen on the top of his hand. "The doctor put my hand flat on the table and hit it hard with a Bible. Then he taped a nickel on it. The wen was gone in a week and a half."

Milkweed. Some had used the milkweed plant to get rid of their warts. When the stalk of one of these plants is broken, drops of white juice form on the severed area. This thick, milky substance was applied to the warts two or three times a day until the warts were gone.

Castor oil. A number of people rubbed castor oil on their warts several times a day until they disappeared. A man from Winchester, New Hampshire, recalled using it on his livestock.

I would bring the colts in in the fall and sometimes they would have warts on their noses. I would rub castor oil on them often, and that would take 'em off.

Other approaches. A piece of silk thread or a horse hair was sometimes used to remove a wart.

Tie a silk thread around the wart. Pull it tight. Leave the thread on and pull it tighter each day. The thread would go through it and the wart would come off in a few days.

———

When I had a big wart, I tied a horse hair around it and left it on until the wart came off. Horse hairs are strange; if you put one in water, after a while it looks like it's alive.

In a nursing home in Presque Isle, Maine, I spoke with a mellow old gentleman who explained an unusual wart treatment.

When I was a boy in school, I had a wart on the back of my hand. One of the boys said he was going to take it off me. He gathered a bunch of spider webs and rolled them up in a little lump the size of a pea. Then he had another boy hold my hand down firm on a brick surface so I couldn't move it. He put the wad of webs on the wart and touched a match to it. It made a red-hot coal and cooked the wart off.

This man proceeded to show me a small scar from this incident, which had taken place over seventy years ago.

In southeastern New Hampshire I spoke with an active eighty-seven-year-old Mohawk medicine woman. She was a short wisp of a thing with poor hearing.

A woman came to me with both hands covered with warts—there must have been ten warts on each hand. I would have had her squeeze milkweed on the warts several times a day, but it was the end of winter and you couldn't get any yet. I told her to take one pound of Epsom salts and boil it hard in a half gallon of water, then let it sit overnight. Each morning she was to take a spoonful of the scum that had formed on top and swallow it; she could follow it with a glass of juice or something. You take it each morning until the warts are gone. A few weeks later, she came back to see me and they were gone.

CHAPPED HANDS

Mutton tallow and lanolin. Some people rubbed chapped or "cracked" hands with mutton tallow. It was made by melting down fat from sheep. To mask the offensive odor, lemon juice was sometimes mixed in with it. Lanolin, which is obtained from the wool of sheep, was used in the same manner. It has a murky yellow color, it is quite sticky, and it does not become rancid.

One woman went right to the source for her lanolin.

> *My folks had thirty-two sheep and it was my job to shear them. I got*
> *blisters whenever I worked at it too long. I would pop the blisters and*
> *grab a sheep and cover my hands with lanolin. I did it every time I went*
> *into the barn. It heals the blisters right up. It's also good for calluses. You*
> *rub it on—it's so soft.*

Urine. Another treatment used for chapped hands was one's own urine. The hands were covered with fresh urine and left to air-dry. Some of the people that had used this treatment spoke quite highly of it. One man recalled, "In school, the nuns used to tell us to use urine when our hands were chapped. This worked when lotions failed." Another man said that his father worked outdoors in a lumberyard all his life. "When my hands got real chapped, he said to urinate on them. It worked right away."

HIVES

Baking soda. Many people treated hives by putting a few good handfuls of baking soda in warm bathwater; this helped to stop the itching. An added benefit was that it cleaned really well; it took off all the old, dry skin.

POISON IVY

Sweet fern. Many people I interviewed had used sweet fern to deal with poison ivy. This "fern" is actually a shrub, *Comptonia peregrina;* one to five feet high, it has a fernlike foliage but looks like a miniature tree. The mature leaves are a dark forest green; when bruised, they give off a sweet, refreshing odor.

A strong tea was made by simmering the leaves and flowering tops of the plant until the water turned dark green. When the tea cooled, the liquid was dabbed on; the treatment was repeated several times a day. For severe cases, a clean rag was dunked in the tea, wrapped around the poisoned area, and left to set. One had to be careful, because the tea stained clothing an earthy, light green.

Sometimes we can get a better idea of how a substance worked by comparing its various uses. The following information points to the conclusion that sweet fern is an excellent disinfectant.

> *Sometimes an old cider or vinegar barrel smelled like an outhouse*
> *unless you left two or three gallons of cider in the bottom of each barrel.*
> *You couldn't use it without spoiling whatever you were going to put into*

it. *To clean it out, I would make sweet-fern tea and leave it to soak. It disinfects and sweetens the barrel.*

You can also take a couple of hoops off the barrel and get the head off. Then take a bunch of dried sweet fern and light it in the barrel; smoke the barrel with it.

Yellow soap. When people mentioned using yellow soap, they were referring to coarse homemade soap or to Fels Naptha, a brand of laundry soap. Yellow soap was lathered on poison ivy and left to dry. The treatment was repeated several times a day. A few people told me that this would dry up the poison and keep the rash from spreading.

Plantain. Some favored plantain leaves.

If shredded and kneaded until juicy, plantain quickly deals with poison ivy and poison oak that can't be treated by any other means. Place the bruised leaves on the poison ivy and bandage them on; leave them on for a day.

Baking soda. To ease ivy poisoning, some had taken a bath with a cup of baking soda added to the water. A baking-soda paste was also used. One man gave his recollection of the process: "Make a plaster of baking soda and water. Dip gauze in the plaster and apply to the affected area. Do this a few times a day."

An area that had a lot of poison ivy in it was on fire. My boy was near there and he breathed in the fumes. He had poison ivy so bad that I had to bathe him with baking-soda water every fifteen minutes.

Other approaches. A paste of Epsom salts and water was applied to the poisoned area. Kerosene was sometimes dabbed on. The area was soaked in a solution of chlorine bleach and water. The celandine and jewelweed plants were also used; either plant would be bruised until juicy, and rubbed over the affected area.

We used to live by the creek, so we had our share of poison ivy. We'd take the jewelweed plant, all but the roots, and squanch it up in our hands. We'd roll it back and forth to get the juice out of it. Then we'd rub the juice over the rash. The stem is transparent with a kind of green juice—we'd make whistles out of them when we were kids. The plant has green things that look like little bananas: you touch them and they break into seeds. My friend had poison ivy on her face and she went to the doctor's, then ended up treating it with jewelweed. If you know you're going to be around poison ivy, you use that first and you won't get it.

ATHLETE'S FOOT

Athlete's foot is a harmless fungal infection, but often it is most annoying. Because the fungus in question incubates and thrives in moisture, the old-time treatment is still good advice.

> *Wash your feet twice a day, change your socks twice a day, and wash the insides of your shoes every other day. Every time you wash your feet, rub cornstarch on them. It will dry the moisture and heal the feet.*

> *My feet were like a half-cooked piece of meat and real smelly. I went to an old horse doctor that they wouldn't take a dead cat to. He told me to keep my feet dry, especially between the toes. It worked and I haven't had it since.*

Other advice included putting on clean white socks, because the dye in colored socks can be irritating, and rotating pairs of shoes, giving each pair a full twenty-four hours to dry.

Foot soaks. Some people soaked their feet at least once a day in a tub of hot water with Epsom salts added to it. One man claimed that salt-pork brine was the best thing. Others chose to bleach out the fungus by soaking their feet daily in a tub of hot water with chlorine bleach in it (a quarter-cup of bleach to a quart of water).

Manure and urine. For stubborn cases of athlete's foot, and for other foot problems, manure or urine often brought good results.

> *Years ago, during the summer months, my feet would get real bad. They would bleed, stink, and ooze; I used to hop around with the pain. I tried all the commercial athlete's-foot preparations that were available, but nothing worked. An old Indian—I think Tommy Owl was his name—told me to urinate on my feet for several days in a row.*
>
> *I went into the shower and urinated on my feet, covered them real good, and didn't rinse them off. Then I let my feet air-dry. I did this for three days in a row and my athlete's foot cleared up and I haven't had it since.*

> *My feet used to stink so bad that I had to wash them and change my socks four times a day. When I went to a movie I would put my feet way back under the seat so the person that sat in back of me would think it was their feet that smelled. But I learned what to do: throughout the day I saved my urine in a pail and I soaked my feet with it. I'd do this about three days in a row and it would take care of the odor for about a month.*

When we were growing up, I had a bad case of athlete's foot: my skin
was badly cracked and always irritated. An old Indian told me to find a
pasture with fresh cow manure in it and walk barefoot through every
cowflop I could find. I was told to do this three or four times a day for ten
days and then to come back and see him.

Ten days later my feet were normal again and I paid the old Indian a
visit. He told me I wouldn't get it again as long as I lived.

—

My father learned how to cure his feet from the Indians. If he had
corns, calluses, or athlete's foot, he would stand in a manure pile for one
hour every other day for a week because it cured the feet. After each treat-
ment he would soak his feet in Epsom salt and hot water.

Gout is, of course, another topic, but the following story indicates that this "foot
treatment" was used on other conditions too.

Cow manure is good for gout. Harry came over to the house and asked
if we minded if he stayed until the cow had a bowel movement. He stepped
into it while it was still hot to draw the inflammation out.

From reading "The Song of Songs" in *The Midrash Rabbah*, one learns not only that
the cow-manure treatment was practiced on another continent, but that it was once considered a simple and sure cure. In discussing the ease of redemption, a teacher describes
"a man who suffered with his feet and who went round to all the doctors and could not
find a cure, till at last one came and said to him, 'If you want to be cured, there is a very
easy way of doing it; plaster your feet with the excrement of cattle.'" [1]

CORNS AND CALLUSES

Foot soaks. A corn or a callus is usually caused by wearing shoes that don't fit properly; when the shoe irritates the foot, a hard lump is formed. A common treatment (which
some still practice) was to soak the foot well, often with Epsom salts in the water, and
then to scrape or whittle the softened corn off the skin.

Grandma used to soak her feet in hot water and then file her corns
with a steel rasp. If they bled or anything, or if she thought it was going to

[1] H. Freedman, B.A., Ph.D., and Maurice Simon, M.A., transl. and ed., *The Midrash Rabbah*, vol. 4, (London, Jerusalem, and New York: Soncino Press, 1977), p. 100.

be real sore, she put turpentine on it.

Castor oil. Unfortunately, sometimes soaking and scraping were not enough. One treatment that some reported to be highly effective was to rub a corn or callus with castor oil two or three times a day.

> *I had a callus on the bottom of my foot and it was so sore. At the time*
> *I had a broken hip and I couldn't bend over. I put castor oil on a face cloth*
> *and rubbed the foot on the cloth each morning and night. In four or five*
> *days it was gone.*

Another approach. A man from Walpole, New Hampshire, explained a rather unusual method he had used.

> *Take four white fish-shell buttons and the juice of one lemon. Soak the*
> *buttons in the juice overnight; it will melt the buttons and turn them into*
> *a cream-like salve. If the buttons are not real fish-shell, they will not melt.*
> *I would apply it twice a day for a few days and the corns would fall off.*

MISCELLANEOUS FOOT CONDITIONS

A BLACK-AND-BLUE NAIL

Piercing. When a toenail or a fingernail had been injured and there was blood trapped underneath it, some people pierced the nail to relieve the pressure and thus put an end to the pain. A woman who had grown up on a large Connecticut farm recalled the treatment.

> *A horse stepped on my foot. My toenail turned black-and-blue and got*
> *bloody underneath. My husband took a paper clip (any item with a blunt*
> *end will do) and heated it well with a match. He put the hot end of the clip*
> *over the bruised area and burnt a small hole in the nail. The blood came*
> *out and that relieved the pressure: the nail stopped aching. It sure hurt*
> *when he did it, but only for an instant.*

INGROWN TOENAILS

Lifting. A man explained a simple treatment for an ingrown toenail.

> *Take a piece of wool yarn and see-saw it under the corner of the toe-*
> *nail—work it like floss. Get the yarn as deep and far down as you can.*
> *Snip the ends of the yarn and leave it in. It would make the corner of the*
> *nail grow upwards instead of down into your skin.*

LICE

Body lice make their home in the hair and clothing. They are difficult to eradicate because they produce a strong gluelike substance to attach their eggs ("nits") to the hair.

Kerosene. In the old days, kerosene was the standard treatment used to get rid of head lice. It was poured into the hair, and the head was wrapped in a towel for an hour or two before it was washed out. While the kerosene was still in, a fine-toothed comb was used to loosen the eggs.

A lady with lots of kindly character written on her face spoke to me in a near-whisper; she was reluctant to tell the following story:

> When I was in the second grade, the girl that sat in front of me in school had a part down the middle of her head. I would sit there fascinated, watching the bugs in that part. Often, the teacher couldn't get my attention.
>
> Well, it wasn't long before I caught them. My mother kept me home from school, sopped my head with kerosene, and left that on for a few hours. My nosy old aunt lived nearby and knew I was home—she came over to see what was wrong. She could smell it as soon as she walked in the door. I was so embarrassed.

In Winsted, Connecticut, a lady explained how her family had avoided head lice.

> Every Saturday morning it was a ritual to soak the head in kerosene and wrap it with a towel. We'd leave it on for an hour, then we'd wash it out with yellow soap. If you left it on too long, it would burn and you would lose your hair. One man lost it and never got it back.

———

> I went to my hairdresser in '47 and told her I had some kind of disease: the back of my neck was all broken out. She raised my hair and said, "You won't believe this, but you're lousy!" (I'd tried on bathrobes about a week before; that's probably where I got them.)
>
> She put kerosene on my hair and had me go outdoors in the yard for about an hour and a half. She didn't want anyone to know; she thought they wouldn't come to her place again because they'd be afraid of catching lice.
>
> I was a teacher and I went to work after I left there. The receptionist said to me, "Hey, you got your hair done! How nice and alive it looks!" I'd just come from all those lice. I looked at her and thought how strange it was she had used that word "alive." But she looked so innocent. [A few sources did mention that the "oil treatment" gave the hair a certain vitality and luster.]

A couple of folks told me that the kerosene could make a person bald if left on the head too long. In Hinsdale, Massachusetts, a spirited Yankee claimed that this was a fact horse thieves had learned to take advantage of.

> *Years back, if you found a man with your horse, you could shoot him on the spot; it was the law, there was no argument. When you stole a man's horse, you would take kerosene oil and rub it in good over an area of its body to change the markings. You'd leave it on and in a couple of days it would blister and take the hair off. Then the new hair would grow in white. A few weeks later, you could take the horse out of hiding and sell it in the same area.*

Other approaches. Occasionally, the head was doused with vinegar. Two people recalled unusual head-lice treatments.

> *I grew up in a small town. In this particular town, selectmen, assessors, and overseers of the poor were all the same. They saw to it that the poor got food, different people provided wood—the town paid for a lot of it. My father was a selectman, and when the poor had cooties, he would go to their homes and shave their heads.*

—

> *Whenever I had lice, Father would steep tobacco leaves, take the leaves out, and douse my head with the solution. He'd put a bandanna over it and leave it on overnight. He'd shampoo my head in the morning.*

Influenza and Fevers

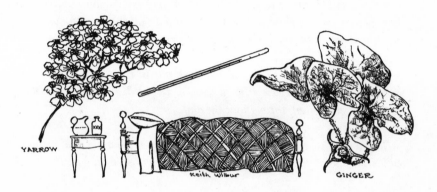

YARROW   keith wilbur   GINGER

In the 1500s, the Italians were plagued with an infectious disease that they called influenza; this name was chosen because they believed it was caused by the influence of the stars.[1] In the 1700s, the French named it *La Grippe;* the origin of the word means "to take hold of."

There were times when I asked people what they had done to treat influenza and a troubled expression came over their faces. A brawny backwoods man who is now confined to a wheelchair summed up the confusion nicely, "There *is* no cure for influenza: It takes so many days to come on, so many days to get better, and so many days to go."

Old-time treatment involved consuming large quantities of fluids, and going to bed and adding extra blankets. Many took a laxative. Some seniors recalled that old adage, "Feed a cold and starve a fever." According to some Yankees, years ago, influenza was called a "hard cold," and indeed, many similarities in treatment can be seen.

[1] Thomas Faulkner, A.M., Ph.D., M.D., and J. H. Charmichael, A.M., M.D., *The Cottage Physician* (Springfield, Mass.: King, Richardson & Co., 1894), p. 208.

In *American Indian Medicine,* Virgil Vogel writes that Native Americans dealt with fevers in a similar manner: "Indian fever treatment commonly included rest, sweating, purgation, and a liquid diet or no food at all, in addition to the antifever medicines."[2]

Alcohol. Some seniors felt that various types of alcohol, especially whiskey, were effective for treating influenza and fevers brought on by other causes.

> *Take lemonade and a huge shot of whiskey, as hot as you can drink it, a hot shower, and go right to bed. Cover up with all the blankets you can find. It will get the blood circulating and warm up the whole system.*

> *Start with a bottle of bourbon whiskey; put in rock candy, raw cherries, and orange peel. Leave it for a week or two. When you have a fever, take a large gulp often, throughout the day.*

> *Take a glass of good, fortified wine, add honey and lemon, and bring it to a boil. It makes you sweat like a horse and brings everything out.*

> *Put into a jar one pint of rum, seven ounces of glycerine, and ten ounces of honey. Shake it up good and take a spoonful as needed.*

Onions. Some people sliced an onion and secured it around the neck; others took onion syrup. One woman told me that whenever she had the flu she would chop up an onion, put it on a plate, and sleep beside it. "I always thought it worked," she said. Onions were secured to other areas of the body as well.

> *Bind slices of raw onion on the tops and bottoms of the wrists; also the balls of the feet. Leave them on all night and repeat in the morning. Continue the treatment until the fever goes away.*

> *Take slices of onions and heat them in the wood ashes on the stove. Put them in a cloth and place that on the forehead. It will bring the fever down.*

Herbal teas. Many seniors felt that inducing perspiration with herbal teas was an effective treatment for influenza and fevers. The most popular of these teas was ginger.

> *When we were sick, my mother would wrap us up in a special old robe and put lots of blankets on us. She'd give us a cup of ginger tea, more if we were real sick. Best thing in the world that I know of. You would sweat your eyeballs out.*

---

[2] Virgil J. Vogel, *American Indian Medicine,* (Norman, Okla.: University of Oklahoma Press, 1970), p. 205.

When my husband had the flu or a cold, I would give him a few cups of ginger tea to warm him up—and did it ever! I would have to change the sheets, because they would be wet from perspiration.

Some favored yarrow:

Yarrow is very bitter. Steep it and add sugar. We took it for any ailment. When my baby had scarlet fever, Grandma came over and put yarrow under the sheet of the crib and gave the baby a little yarrow tea every few hours.

—

Yarrow grows wild; there used to be millions of plants all over the place. You cut the plants and hang them somewhere to dry—but don't touch the blossoms. When you get the grippe, cut off some of the blossoms and steep them until the color comes out. You have to add sugar because a strong cup is bitter as hell. If someone has a fever, I personally guarantee it will break it up overnight: it really makes you perspire. You drink a few good swallows at a time throughout the day, and you must go to bed. You will be back to normal the next day.

Yarrow was used by the American Indians. As a fever treatment, some took it internally and others burned the flowers and breathed in the fumes. One tribe would burn the flowers to revive a comatose person. [3]

Catnip and camomile teas were also taken for influenza and fevers.

Other approaches. Some had soaked the feet in mustard water, others had taken a mustard-water bath. Baking-soda baths were taken. Cold water and ice were used in various applications: a cold cloth or ice was applied to the back of the neck; a cold pack was placed on the forehead; a person was immersed in cold water; a cold compress was placed on the lower legs; a cold compress was placed on each arm where the elbows bend. Some had taken a sponge bath with rubbing alcohol; others had put rubbing alcohol on various parts of the body.

[3] Vogel, op.cit., p. 397.

- 10 -

Problems of Infancy and Childhood

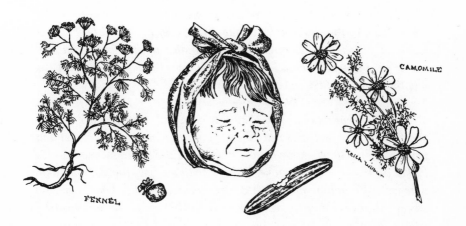

PREMATURE BABIES

Most people with premature babies treated them in similar fashion; even phrases used to express how small they were often echoed one another.

Tiny babies were never washed with soap until they became stronger; instead, they were rubbed down with oil—usually olive oil. Also, it was important to make an incubator of sorts.

Warm up bricks or rocks in the oven and wrap them in flannel. Put them around the baby in a crib. Don't fondle the baby, and don't diaper it, just put a rag under it.

—

I was born early, I weighed three pounds. I'm told I was put in a rocking chair in front of the oven. Father made a roaring fire and I was half-baked.

—

My brother was born in 1915, in the seventh month. He was wrapped in cotton and placed in a dresser drawer that had been padded very well. He had no fingernails, no hair. Hot water bottles were tucked in around him.

———

I was born two and a half pounds. Grandma used a teacup to make a bonnet to fit me. Put me in the oven, laid on cotton. She cleaned me with olive oil to strengthen me. I was too delicate to dress.

———

The neighbors' baby was born weighing two pounds. The doctors said she would die. You could slip a wedding ring over her wrist. Doll clothes wouldn't fit, she was so tiny. She was bundled up in flannel and kept warm in a shoebox behind the stove. She was never washed for six months. Well, she lived to be an old lady.

———

In my seventh month, my baby was born and weighed three pounds and four ounces; and she lived. She slept all the time. I took a basket and placed cotton flannel on the bottom to make a little mattress, and kept the basket on the back of the stove. Fed her with an eye dropper; milk with lime water [from limestone] in it. I never washed her, but I oiled her with sweet oil once a day to keep the heat in. She grew to be a healthy adult—although she was always small. She died a few years ago from a heart ailment.

———

My brother weighed a little over two pounds when he was born. He was so little, they put him in a shoebox and kept him very warm near the stove. Born in September, in the seventh month. He was coal black because of lack of oxygen, and he stayed that way for a day and a half. He was carried on a pillow, of course.

He is now sixty-five, healthy all his life. He went through the war. And he's never been sick like the rest of us.

UMBILICAL HERNIA

Flannel belly bands. In order to keep a newborn from developing a herniated navel, a flannel belly band was wrapped around the infant's stomach and abdomen and secured snugly on the side. They were made between four and six inches wide, and the cloth was sometimes feather-stitched so it wouldn't ravel. Sometimes they were decorated with fancy, bright-colored embroidery. Most people kept them on their babies until they were five or six months old, some less. Although one lady commented that belly bands were "good for nothing, because they were constantly wet, especially with a baby boy," many felt they were a "definite must."

In many cases it worked real good. When the baby coughed, the navel stuck out more. Push the belly button back in and put a copper penny over it, and the band over that. A baby had to be a few days old before you used the penny. The band would go on as soon as they were born.

———

We felt it was dangerous not to use them, because if a baby strained it might get a hernia, especially a boy baby. I kept my son in them for the longest time. They used to be tied by three little strings about the size of tape.

———

Belly bands were twelve inches wide and then doubled over—they covered pretty near the whole stomach. Part of their purpose was to keep babies warm—grandmothers still think you have to keep a baby's tummy and back warm.

———

I've made a good many belly bands. They had little gussets in them so they'd fit right around the tummy. When my little boy was a few days old, the navel was starting to pop out. My sister-in-law brought over a silver dollar with a hole punched in it: it was placed over the navel to keep it from turning into a "breach." The band went on over that. We used flannel outing; it was light and soft.

———

My little grandson is fourteen months old. When he says, "What's that?" and points to his protruding navel, I say, "It's something that's not supposed to be there." Now the doctor says it's a hernia and it'll disappear in time. If he'd had a belly band, he would be OK.

COLIC

Fennel. Weak fennel tea was often chosen as a remedy for colicky babies. It was made by boiling half a teaspoon of fennel seeds in a cup of water for about five minutes.

Fennel tea is the best thing in the world for babies with colic. Boil a few seeds in water and make a mild solution, strain it, let it cool, and add a little sugar. Put it in a bottle. You don't have to burp a child on the shoulder so much when you give it to a baby.

Fennel is a cousin to caraway. An Italian woman taught me how to make spaghetti sauce from scratch—taught me to put some fennel in the sauce to move gas and add flavor.

———

I made fennel-seed tea for a baby's bellyache. The poor little fellows would pull their knees up to their chests and screech. I strained out the seeds and fed the tea to my babies with a spoon. (I didn't have bottles because I breast-fed.) It was soothing to the stomach and it would break up the gas.

A hospitable lady from Storrs, Connecticut, had used fennel in a different manner:

We would save old linen napkins, we never threw them away. We would put a piece of bread into a scrap of old linen and tie it into a little pouch. Then we'd dunk the pouch in fennel tea and squeeze the bag to make a dough and get the excess moisture out. Whenever one of my babies had colic, I would give him one of those to chew on.

Fennel-and-catnip tea. Some of the people with whom I spoke had given a tea of fennel and catnip to colicky babies. One lady told me, "Steep catnip and fennel, then strain it. You judge the strength by the smell and taste. Babies like it, it's calming and soothing."

Camomile tea. Others had preferred to deal with colic by giving the baby camomile tea.

Camomile tea was always kept in a pot on the stove. It's excellent for babies with colic. Between feedings, give them a bottle with camomile tea in it mixed with a teaspoon of corn syrup. It would keep them from having bowel problems.

DIAPER RASH

Cornstarch. By far the most popular remedy for diaper rash was cornstarch—which now happens to be making a comeback as a baby powder. The baby's bottom was powdered with it each time the diaper was changed. Many used it on a regular basis instead of commercial products. One woman's sentiments were shared by several others.

Baby powder was too expensive, so we always used cornstarch. Anyway, it worked better than any type of medication or powder you could buy—it was the best.

———

Cornstarch is excellent for diaper rash, itching, and bedsores. I used to work for a doctor who used it on so many things. It would clear a diaper rash up in no time. And he never had a patient with a bedsore.

A couple variations include cornstarch mixed with a little lard, and equal parts of flour and cornstarch mixed together.

Browned flour. A number of grandmothers believed that when a diaper rash got out of hand, browned flour worked the best. An energetic lady recalled the time that her baby's rash turned into blisters.

My baby had blisters on his bottom from a urine burn, a raw bottom. I couldn't set the kid on the floor, he was crazy with the rash. The doctor gave me a salve to rub on the butt. You can't put a salve on a raw bottom! The kid would scream—a blistered butt can't be rubbed.

The neighbor gave me a remedy: put flour in a pie plate on the stove until it browns well. Keep shaking the plate so it doesn't burn. When it's dark brown, put it in a jar. Dab it on, powder the baby good with it. Use it each time you change the diaper. It's the most fantastic thing—even if the skin was blistered, it would cure it.

Some had scorched the flour in the oven. In either case, the effect was the same—it formed a seal that protected the baby's bottom from urine.

Other approaches. In some households, baking soda was applied each time a baby's diaper was changed.

A lady from Little Falls, New York, had witnessed the curative properties of plantain in her earlier years.

The minister's wife had twins, and she died a few weeks later. When they were a month old, an aunt took each one. But they had been born so unhealthy they looked just like little old men. Grandma was asked if she would take them, and she ended up having them for seven and a half years. They were so sickly, and their bottoms were real sore.

I had to go out and pick plantain leaves and wash them and chop them up. Grandma put them in the diaper each time she changed them. It took a few days to heal their bottoms.

When they grew up, they both became ministers.

———

Diaper rash often came from diapers that weren't clean. Boil diapers and dry them in the sunshine to kill the germs. It will clear it up right away.

MEASLES AND CHICKEN POX

Warmth. Our elders knew there was nothing capable of killing the virus outright once a child became infected with measles or chicken pox. With measles, the treatment involved controlling the course of the disease. The first consideration was to "keep the child warm to bring the measles out," as it was believed that "if they didn't blossom well, they would break out on the inside and make the child deathly ill."

> *For measles, give the child a good hot bath to bring them out. They pop up quick after a hot bath. Then put a flannel nightshirt on the child. Roll him up in a blanket—the heat makes it all come out.*

———

> *My son had measles in the stomach and he felt awful. I gave him hot lemonade and made him sit behind the hot stove to keep good and warm so they would blossom. He began to sweat and feel better when they came out.*

———

> *Got to keep a child warm to bring out measles. If you don't, the measles cannot come out freely. They would break out on the inside. Give the child hot drinks. When you got the measles to come out, the fever would go down.*

———

> *Grandma lived practically next door to us and I stayed with her a lot. She used to sleep in little white bonnets with fancy lace to keep her ears warm. She made me sleep in one too, even in the summer. When I had the measles, she wrapped a hot brick in a towel and put it on my feet. When the brick lost its heat, she put in another one: said it was very important to keep me warm. I wish I'd saved one of those lace bonnets.*

Baking soda. For both measles and chicken pox, a popular treatment to control the itching involved baking soda. For measles, a baking-soda bath was the most likely remedy; for chicken pox, it was a baking-soda paste dabbed on the sores. However, there was some crossover.

> *Put a good handful of baking soda in the bathwater and bathe the child in it. It brings the measles out, stops itching, and brings the fever down. Do it whenever they start itching.*

———

> *For chicken pox, put about a cup of baking soda in a few cups of water. Sponge the child with it so the soda dries on. It's to keep the child from scratching the eruptions—almost impossible to do, except the bicarbonate of soda relieved it some.*

———

A soda-water bath—a regular bath, not a soak—would stop the itch when a child had measles or chicken pox. I would do it three or four times a day. Also, give a hot drink such as ginger, sage, or catnip tea.

———

Wasn't much you could do for chicken pox. Give the child warm liquids. Make sure he doesn't scratch. Make a baking-soda paste and dab it on the sores—it stops the itching.

Some children with measles complain that light hurts their eyes; from this came the false notion that exposure to light during the infection could damage the eyes or cause blindness. Many seniors recalled being kept in a dark room for the duration of the illness: shades were drawn and sometimes heavy material was tacked over the windows. One lady remembered, "Mother covered my eyes with gauze all the while I had the measles. She was afraid I'd go blind."

If chicken pox are scratched, scars may result. Mittens or socks were sometimes put on the child's hands to prevent scratching.

Manure. Sometimes sheep manure or goat manure was steeped and drunk as a tea for measles that wouldn't come out. A heavyset Vermont lady had almost experienced a variation of the treatment: "When I had the measles, they wanted to give me sheep pills and cider." She quizzed me in a deep voice, "You know what that is, don't you?" Another Yankee recalled taking "sheep shit and syrup."

The goat-manure tea was often referred to as "nanny tea." A man said bluntly, "We dragged measles out with nanny-turd tea." One person called it "nanny-plum tea."

Other approaches. I received one remedy that called for taking a teaspoon of goat's urine, "If you're real sick and the measles won't come out." To control the itch of chicken-pox eruptions, some dabbed on various oils such as castor oil or petroleum jelly.

MUMPS

Scarf. I collected little material on the treatment of mumps. Sometimes a scarf was wrapped around the child's head (it was often tied on the top), "to keep the area warm." Flannel was often chosen because it locked in the heat.

Other approaches.

When we had a new baby, we saved the umbilical cord. If anyone had the mumps, we tied a piece of the cord on the child's neck. We saved it for the boys, because mumps in boys is especially dangerous. [It can cause sterility.]

———

Rub sardine grease all over the face and neck, and eat the sardines—I can't eat them to this day. The way we'd tell if we had the mumps was to eat a sour pickle. If you could eat it you didn't have the mumps, because the sourness would make the jaws tighten up, sort of a tension in the jaws.

Another source said to tie raw herring around the neck.

11

Female Concerns

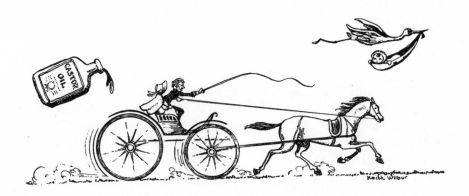

MENSTRUAL CRAMPS AND IRREGULARITIES

Ginger tea. Ginger tea was the most popular remedy for easing the pain of menstrual cramps. Usually a scant teaspoon of powdered ginger was mixed in a cup of hot water, and two or three cups would be taken a day, as needed. Some cut the strong ginger taste with a little milk and sugar, and some used all milk instead of water.

A grandmother explained that ginger tea used to be her old standby.

When I had bad cramps, my mother would give me a large bowl of ginger tea and make me drink the whole thing. It worked well; it would heat the stomach and take the cramps away.

Others likewise mentioned that ginger, a "hot" spice, would "warm the stomach." It was believed that the heat the ginger produced would expand the blood vessels and relax the uterus.

Heat. Some women placed a hot-water bottle over the abdomen; hot baths were taken; one woman mentioned drinking large quantities of hot water. Others felt that a "good hot foot soak" relaxed the uterine muscle; sometimes a tablespoon or two of dry mustard was dissolved in the water.

Pennyroyal tea. Another way to ease menstrual cramps was to drink pennyroyal tea. The dried leaves and flowering tops were steeped in hot water; two or three cups were consumed a day.

Women in the Northeast also used pennyroyal tea for "suppressed menses." According to a number of grandmothers, this term meant cramping without bleeding.

Alcohol. Some women took a good shot of alcohol to relieve cramps, and it didn't seem to matter what kind it was. One source told me that "a good portion of straight gin heats your blood and makes it flow better."

Another grandmother told me that she used to suffer agonizing cramps.

> I would go to the store and buy a package of mixed spices; they would come in a little bag. Mother would take a jug of whiskey and dump just a little out, and put the spices in the bottle. When I had bad cramps, she would give me a jigger. The whiskey tasted like spice and it really did help the cramps.

Other approaches. Other treatments for menstrual cramps were wintergreen tea, peppermint tea, willow-bark tea, and very small quantities of tansy tea. To induce the period when it was late, feet were soaked in hot mustard water. Cinnamon tea was used to curb excessive bleeding.

A Native American told me what the women of his tribe had used for excessive menstrual bleeding.

> Yarrow is a squaw weed—it's the biggest thing that stanches blood. It's good for internal bleeding of almost any kind. A woman with a long period would take a few cups of the tea during her period, or at the beginning for an easier time.

LABOR

Castor oil. The anxiety of not knowing when a baby would arrive could be taxing— particularly when help had to be summoned from a distance and could not stay indefinitely. Our grandmothers had one standard remedy that was used to induce labor when the due date had been reached. The remedy was simply a large dose of castor oil (an ounce or two) mixed with something to cut the taste. A woman was also advised to take castor oil at the first sign of labor "to hurry you along."

The years had gently woven a matrix of wrinkles into the face of a woman I interviewed in Winchester, New Hampshire. She recalled an incident when castor oil had induced labor and brought the baby out quickly.

My sister Arlene and her girlfriend Glenda got pregnant around the same time. The first thing on a Saturday morning in April, Arlene had her baby. Glenda wanted to have her baby on the same day. When I told her about the new arrival, she said, "Arlene isn't going to beat me by much." An old lady had told her that when the baby was due she should take two ounces of castor oil, and that's what she was determined to do. I told her I didn't think it was a good idea, but she wouldn't listen.

Later that day, Glenda was taking a shortcut through the field. My husband looked out the window and said, "God, Glenda's down on the ground hanging on to her stomach." We barely got her to the hospital on time. When they were prepping her, they nearly shaved the baby's head.

She delivered seven hours after she took the castor oil. Apparently it didn't hurt her or the baby, but she was weak from so many bowel movements.

———

I was two weeks overdue and Mother gave me a dose of straight castor oil; a while later, she put me in the car and took me out in the country around the hills on dirt roads. She'd just go boom, *fast, over the bumps and say, "That's the way to go." I went into labor in the car, and Mother rushed me to the hospital. I was there about four hours before my daughter was born. She weighed six pounds, seven and a half ounces.*

———

My baby was supposed to be due on the tenth of March. This old lady said to take a dose of castor oil. I took it and went to bed. Nothing happened until about eleven o'clock that night. I woke up and had bad labor pains; the physic was working.

I was in agony. My poor husband was trying to put my stockings on to get me dressed to go to the hospital. I almost had the baby in the toilet because the pains were coming so fast. We barely made it to the hospital on time. They gave me ether because the baby was coming so fast they were afraid I would be torn.

Physicians also used castor oil to speed up labor and control the time of birth.

My doctor was leaving for Europe and it was about time for me to have my baby. He gave me four tablespoons of castor oil with root beer, and it did the trick. I spent a lot of time admiring the plumbing that day. I took it Saturday around noon and I started labor that evening. I delivered Sunday night. It physicked you so hard that the pressure would make you begin labor.

———

I was a nurse in a doctor's office, and this woman was three weeks overdue and very uncomfortable. The doctor had me give her some castor oil and grape juice—it was the most God-awful-looking stuff you ever saw—a greenish, vile color. The lady threw it up, but she begged for more. The doctor agreed to it, so I gave her another dose. Two hours later, she went into labor, and she was very grateful.

Some seniors told me they had used castor oil without success. They said that it didn't work unless it was taken in a large dose, near or beyond the due date.

URINARY-TRACT INFECTIONS

Cream of tartar. Cream of tartar was often used to treat infections of the urinary tract—a small teaspoon would be stirred in a glass of water. Some chose to add lemon juice or a sweetener. Two or three glasses would be taken a day, and the treatment continued for a day or two after symptoms disappeared. Several people reported that this treatment would give relief in one or two days.

Grandmothers spoke of the treatment and variations.

When I worked in the paper mill I got an infection. I was always going to the bathroom to urinate, but only a few drops would come out at a time. I kept running back and forth. I had to go home because I was holding up production. Mother gave me cream of tartar in water a few times and it cleared it up.

———

Pregnant women with urinary problems were encouraged to drink cream of tartar in water—it clears the kidneys right up. We would pour one quart of boiling water over a large tablespoon of cream of tartar. After it settled, we sometimes strained it and then let it cool. We would drink two or three glasses a day until the problem was gone.

———

When I'd get a bladder infection, I would wet my pants, I had to go so bad. I'd mix a half a teaspoon of cream of tartar and a half a teaspoon of baking soda in eight ounces of water (not very cold). I'd take it once a day; it's best in the morning on an empty stomach.

———

Whenever I got a kidney infection or edema, I'd mix a teaspoon of cream of tartar, a teaspoon of sugar, and a few drops of wintergreen oil in a glass of water. Whenever my ankles got bad, I would take that and lose four pounds.

Cream of tartar (tartaric acid) is potassium salt from grape-wine sediment. At the turn of the century, many doctors prescribed two forms of potassium for urinary-tract infections: potash (crude potassium carbonate) and niter, better known as saltpeter (potassium nitrate). A retired nurse proudly recalled the time she was visiting a patient who had not urinated in three days; she gave the woman niter and she voided within half an hour.

Water. There were seniors who had consumed large quantities of water to flush out a urinary infection.

Other approaches. Some drank cranberry juice for urinary-tract infections. I was surprised to learn that, at least among country folks, this treatment was not as popular as it is today. Then I learned that cranberry juice was not a staple in most homes, and for many, trips to the general store were infrequent.

Also used were juniper-berry gin, pumpkin seeds, goldthread tea, asparagus, parsley tea, and mullein tea.

12

Preventive Medicine

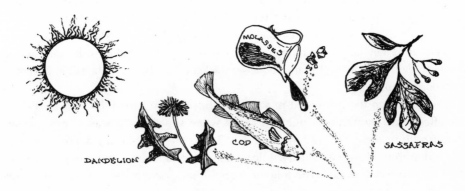

SPRING TONICS

Today's booming health-food industry bears witness to the fact that a large number of people are practicing preventive medicine. This interest in maintaining health is not a new phenomenon: I am amazed at the number of times I began an interview and the first thing that people remembered was sulfur-and-molasses, taken in the spring as a conditioner.

There was good reason for people to take their tonics in the spring. Often winters were harsh, leaving snow piled up against windows and forcing people to stay indoors and inactive. Fresh fruits and vegetables were scarce at this time of year, and diets lacked certain essential nutrients. When spring finally rolled around, there was a need to flow with the vitality of the new season and a need to correct the effects of winter living.

Sulfur. In my entire collection, sulfur-and-molasses is the single most popular remedy. Many seniors said that "Sulfur was good for a spring cleaning." This was due, in part, to its laxative effect. To "clean blood" and "clean house," equal parts of sulfur and molasses were mixed together in a jar. There were a few variations, such as using less sulfur or adding cream of tartar or onions to the concoction. The amount to be ingested depended on the age of the person: Small children were given half a teaspoon a day, adults took a full tablespoon. The mixture was taken in the morning, often for seven days in a row, usually in March. (One lady told me, "We took it as the robins came.") There were some who took it for only a few days and others for as long as two weeks. A lady that grew up in a family of sixteen remembered taking it all through Lent, though the dosage was much smaller than standard. Some people took it three days on, three days off, until they had taken nine doses. A few took it in the fall as well as the spring. One lady claimed that "Sulfur and molasses thickened the blood in the fall and thinned the blood in the spring."

Comments on the sulfur-and-molasses treatment were varied. Because of its laxative effect, one woman was right on target when she said, "It was a spring clean-up—everything went." Many concurred that "it was the worst-tasting damn stuff." One little old grandmother was a real soldier when she said, "You knew it was doing you good, so you didn't mind." The following anecdotes give a better idea of how people felt about it and what its purpose was.

I used to hide under the porch when I saw it coming. It was supposed to give you pep after the winter was over, when you got the blues.

—

Sulfur-and-molasses was supposed to take the poison out of you. We used to line up at the kitchen sink to take it. Father kept it in a pitcher that was like a crock; we each had our own spoon. It kept us from getting sick and it helped to clear up pimples.

—

We took sulfur-and-molasses in the spring to get the winter out of us. When you broke wind, it used to stink. My sister and I went to the store once and she let one go. The clerk turned around and said "What the hell happened here?" We got out of there fast.

—

When I was a young fellow on the farm, my parents had a so-called "spring tonic." When the sap started to run in the trees, my thoughts naturally turned to romance, but my mother's thoughts turned to sulfur-and-molasses. How I hated that stuff! A couple of spoonfuls in the morning was supposed to be good for you. Who knows? Maybe it was. I'm still here.

A few people experienced strange side effects from the sulfur-and-molasses treatment. According to one lady,

After you took it a few times, the sulfur would go right out into your socks. At the end of the day we would shake our socks over the hot wood stove and the flames would make different designs.

The New Dispensatory, written in 1821, supports the validity of the above claim: "It seems to pass through the whole habit, and manifestly transpires through the pores of the skin, as appears from the sulphurous smell of persons who have taken it, and from silver in their pockets imbibing a blackish cast, which is the known effect of sulphurous fumes."[1]

Some people claimed that while they were taking their clothes off at night, the sparks would fly because ingestion of the concoction created static electricity.

There were other ways besides spring tonic to use sulfur for preventive medicine. Some wore dry sulfur bags around their necks to ward off disease. If there was sickness going around, the house might be closed up tight and a sulfur candle lit. Some threw sulfur on the hot stove periodically to fumigate the house. According to one grandmother,

Mother would throw a pinch of sulfur on the stove three or four times a week in the winter. It made a blue blaze that was very entertaining for us.

When our grandparents were growing up, the medical community frequently used sulfur. One medical text reads: "Sulphur is used internally as a laxative, in certain skin diseases, in chronic rheumatism, etc. . . . Applied externally, sulphur is a parasiticide, and is the best remedy for scabies." Further, "When the time comes to disinfect the sickroom, the best agent for the ordinary person is probably sulphur (described by Greek Dioscorides and by Roman Pliny)."[2]

Other tonics used. Some people drank tea made from the rootbark of the sassafras tree as a spring tonic. A cup of this reddish-orange beverage was taken seven to fourteen days in a row, often in March, to clean and thin the blood.

Father and I used to walk down this old dirt road and dig sassafras roots. There was one spot where the trees grew. When we got home, we would peel the bark off the roots and let it dry—it had a wonderful smell.

Father said it made a good health drink, and we all got a cup of tea a couple of times day in the middle of March, for about five days in a row. He also drank the tea when he had problems with his stomach.

Some ate quantities of dandelion greens in the spring, before they got bitter. A few took cream of tartar mixed in water; lemon juice or Epsom salts might be added to the mixture. Some had made concoctions with honey and vinegar.

---

[1] James Thacher, M.D., *The New Dispensatory*, (Boston: Thomas B. Wait, 1821), p. 391.

[2] Victor Robinson, Ph.C., M.D., ed., *The Modern Home Physician* (New York: William H. Wise and Co., 1939), pp. 240, 689.

For a spring tonic, we would mix a tablespoon of honey in a small glass of vinegar to flush out the blood stream. Mother always said that in the winter your blood is heavier. This would flush out impurities that had accumulated over the winter.

COD-LIVER OIL

Many seniors recalled taking cod-liver oil, especially in the cold months; some took it daily, others once or twice a week. The dose varied: a few drops for a baby, a teaspoon for a youngster, up to a full tablespoon for older children and adults. Several people reported that "it was supposed to build you up and make you strong." Some had also taken it to cure illness.

Different seniors gave their recollections of this substance.

In the wintertime at school we were given a whole tablespoon of cod-liver oil every day. It would keep colds away. The government furnished it. You brought your own spoon. At the end of the year the spoon would be green, it was all corroded.

———

Cod-liver oil smelled awful. You'd give it to the baby, a few drops with an eye dropper. You'd give it to them in the morning and you'd smell it on them all day.

———

Cod-liver oil came in a bottle shaped like a fish. We'd get it in school all year around, along with an iodine pill. It was our way of getting vitamins—in the winter we didn't have much in the way of vegetables or sunshine.

———

Mother gave us cod-liver oil when we were kids; we ran away. When I'd take it I'd spit it out; it tastes horrible. It was to keep you from getting rickets.

———

Cod-liver oil was good for colds, TB, or other lung problems. For TB, take it three times a day, one teaspoon each time. You could mix it with honey to make it taste better.

———

It was yellow and it stained clothes. It strengthened your bones when you were small so you wouldn't be bowlegged, and it gave you a push for the summer.

CAMPHOR AND OTHER AROMATICS

Items such as camphor, garlic, and asafoetida were worn on the body as preventive medicine. Of these products, camphor was the most widely used by far.

Camphor. Camphor is a solid gum resin produced from the camphor tree, a large evergreen that grows in warm climates. Small chunks of camphor gum or camphor ice (made chiefly of camphor, white wax, spermaceti, and castor oil) were worn by many in cold weather months to prevent sickness. The usual procedure was to place a chunk of the highly aromatic camphor in a small cloth bag and wear it around the neck. This practice was especially popular in times of epidemics; many people mentioned wearing it during the devastating influenza epidemic of 1918.

> *Every winter my mother would place a piece of camphor in a small cloth bag about one inch square. She would pin the bag inside my long underwear. By the time spring rolled around, it would be all evaporated.*

> —

> *Father insisted, when we were young, that we have these horrible smelly bags of camphor around our necks. Supposed to ward off colds and other problems. Kids would make fun of me at school because I smelled like camphor, but I couldn't take it off.*

> —

> *We used camphor bags to keep colds and flu away. I used to wear one pinned to my bra. I used it until about four years ago when they took it off the market. I put camphor-gum cakes in my dresser drawer so my clothes would absorb it. The doctor said it was a good bet no one would come near me, so I wouldn't catch anything.*

> —

> *In the influenza season, I wore camphor bags. They were about one inch square, worn like a scapular, one in front and one in back. I didn't get no flu.*

> —

> *My mother put camphor and goose grease in a little bag and I wore it around my neck in the winter. Lots of kids wore it in school. It stunk. Many babies wore camphor bags pinned to their undershirts, and some people put camphor bags on babies' cribs.*

One lady told me, "I used to put it in with silver to keep it from tarnishing, and it also kept away fleas and lice." Another source claimed that her two little boys were healthy all the time, but the minute she took off their camphor bags they got the measles.

Was the widespread use of camphor an act of blind faith? Robert Tisserand, in *The Art of Aromatherapy,* speaks of the use of aromatics (including camphor) during the

Black Death plague of the Middle Ages. "Aromatics were the best antiseptics available at the time, and the people knew it. . . . Those in closest contact with aromatics, especially the perfumers, were virtually immune. Since all aromatics are antiseptic, it is likely that many of those used were indeed effective protection against the plague."[3]

Other approaches. A few people recalled wearing an asafoetida bag around the neck in winter to prevent illness. Asafoetida is the gum resin of various oriental plants of the carrot family; its most notable property is its horrendous odor. In our local health-food store, I uncapped a jar of asafoetida and took a deep whiff. It was a mistake I am not likely to repeat.

> *All winter long I wore an asafoetida bag—stinkingest stuff you ever*
> *smelled. Smells like a goddamn fox den. That would keep off the flu and*
> *discourage getting a cold.*

Garlic was sometimes worn about the neck. One woman said, "It will protect you from any disease—polio, too." On occasion it was used to "keep witches away" and "drive off evil spirits."

A few mentioned having worn an onion bag on the neck or chest to prevent sickness.

SUMMER COOLANT, WINTER WARM-UP

Switzel. Our ancestors often worked hard on blazing-hot days, taking in the hay and the like, without the labor-saving equipment farmers have today. To fend off heat prostration, a bucket with a ladle in it was commonly brought out to the workers so they could help themselves to a drink of "switzel." Its purpose was to cool the body down and prevent heat cramps. The ingredients and their proportions varied, but powdered ginger was always included. The following is a typical formula:

> 3 Tbsp. ginger
>
> 1 cup vinegar
>
> 1 gal. water
>
> 2 cups sugar (white or brown) or
> molasses, maple syrup, or honey

Some people included oatmeal in the formula. About a third of the people who gave me switzel recipes did not include vinegar.

---

[3] Robert B. Tisserand, *The Art of Aromatherapy* (New York: Inner Traditions International, 1977), pp. 38–39.

Ginger tea makes you sweat—that's what cools you, you know. It was ginger, sugar, and water. We didn't drink it ice cold; no ice in it—as cold as it came out of the water pump. When we ran after we drank it, we would hear it in our tummies, so we called it rattle-belly.

———

Grandfather used to cut hay by hand and always carried a bottle of switzel. He'd go heavy on the ginger and vinegar. When you drank it, smoke would come out of your nose, eyes, ears, everything.

———

We called switzel "ginger water," "guzzle," and "belly wash." A kettle with a ladle went to the hayfields with a little ice floating in it. It was ginger, maple syrup, vinegar, and water. Vinegar quenched your thirst. You could drink all you wanted and it wouldn't hurt you. Lots of plain water gives you cramps when it's hot out, whereas this was comforting.

———

During the haying months we made ginger water. We mixed it up in a twelve-quart milk pail. The beauty of it was, no matter how hot the day, it never gave pains in the stomach. During haytime, that was the best. Good for the flu, too. Drink a good, strong batch.

A few people had used ginger tea as a "winter warmer," which suggests that this common household spice may have been broadly useful in regulating body temperature. A lady from Plymouth, Massachusetts, recalled:

Sometimes our whole family would take the horse and buggy and go out visiting on a winter evening. Usually we were very cold when we got home and Mother would make us all a hot cup of ginger tea with milk and sugar added to make it taste better—nothing warms you up as well.

Another approach. A few folks mentioned taking cream of tartar with water to offset the effects of hot weather.

When we used to go out haying, I would put a few tablespoons of cream of tartar in a large pitcher of water—enough so the color looks creamy, and I'd add a little sugar. This would cool your system down in hot weather.

———

Dad was a farmer. When he came in overheated, Mother gave him cream of tartar, water, and sugar—it cools your blood down. It didn't make him nauseous like cold water would.

Bibliography

Beach, W., M.D. *The American Practice, Condensed; or, The Family Physician.* New York: James McAlister, 1849.

Boettcher, Helmuth. *Wonder Drugs.* Philadelphia and New York: J.B. Lippincott Co., 1963.

Bryan, Cyril P. *The Papyrus Ebers.* London: Garden City Press, 1930.

Corish, J.L., M.D., ed. *Health Knowledge,* vol. 2. New York: Domestic Health Society, 1924.

Faulkner, Thomas, A.M., Ph.D., M.D., and J. H. Charmichael, A.M., M.D. *The Cottage Physician.* Springfield, Mass.: King, Richardson, & Co., 1894.

Fisher, M.F.K. *A Cordiall Water.* Boston and Toronto: Little, Brown, and Co., 1961.

Freedman, H., B.A., Ph.D., and Maurice Simon, M.A., transl. and ed. *The Midrash Ribbah,* vol. 4. London, Jerusalem, and New York: Soncino Press, 1977.

Gosselin, Robert E., M.D., Ph.D.; Harold C. Hodge, Ph.D., D.Sc.,; et al. *Clinical Toxicology of Commercial Products.* Baltimore: Williams and Wilkins Co., 1977.

Hamilton, Alexander V. *The Household Cyclopedia of Practical Receipts and Daily Wants.* Springfield, Mass.: W.J. Holland and Co., 1874.

Hickernell, Marguerite R., and Ella W. Brewer. *Adam's Herbs, Their Story from Eden On.* Woodstock Vt.: Elm Tree Press, 1947.

Klauber, Laurence M. *Rattlesnakes,* vol. 2. Berkeley and Los Angeles: University of California Press, 1972.

Mitchill, Samuel L., M.D.; James R. Manley, M.D.; Felix Pascalis, M.D.; Charles Drake, M.D. *The Medical Repository on Original Essays and Intelligence,* vol. 6. New York: William A. Mercein, 1821.

Pocumtuc Housewife (The), A Guide to Domestick Cookery, by Several Ladies. Massachusetts: Deerfield Parish Guild, 1805 (reprinted in 1971).

Robinson, Victor, Ph.C., M.D., ed. *The Modern Home Physician.* New York: William H. Wise and Co., 1939.

Scholl, Frank B., Ph.G., M.D., ed. *Library of Health.* Philadelphia: Historical Publishing Co., 1920.

Thacher, James, M.D. *The New Dispensatory.* Boston: Thomas B. Wait, 1821.

Tisserand, Robert B. *The Art of Aromatherapy.* New York: Inner Traditions International, Ltd., 1977.

Vogel, Virgil J. *American Indian Medicine.* Norman: University of Oklahoma Press, 1970.

Wigginton, Eliot, ed. *The Foxfire Book.* New York: Doubleday and Co., 1972.

Yemm, J.R., F.N.A., D.O., N.D., ed. *The Medical Herbalist.* vol. 11. National Association of Medical Herbalists of Great Britain, Ltd., 1937.

If you have remedies to share, please write to:
The Folk Medicine Connection
285 Greenfield Road
Montague, MA 01351

Index